The Empathy Trap: Understanding Antisocial Personalities

Dr Jane McGregor is a freelance writer and trainer, and a part-time lecturer at the Institute of Mental Health, University of Nottingham. Her academic subject area is public health. She holds a PhD in this area, gained at the London School of Hygiene and Tropical Medicine and funded by the Wellcome Trust. Jane previously worked in the NHS and voluntary sector for many years, mostly in the field of addiction treatment, and she has published widely in this area.

Tim McGregor is a freelance consultant, writer and trainer. He is a mental health practitioner of many years' standing and has worked in both the NHS and the UK voluntary sector, most recently as a commissioning advisor. Tim has a keen interest in evidence-based approaches to behaviour change and this forms the foundation of much of his training work. Tim is writing his first novel.

Overcoming Common Problems Series

Selected titles

A full list of titles is available from Sheldon Press,
36 Causton Street, London SW1P 4ST and on our website at
www.sheldonpress.co.uk

Breast Cancer: Your treatment choices
Dr Terry Priestman

Coeliac Disease: What you need to know
Alex Gazzola

**Coping Successfully with Chronic Illness:
Your healing plan**
Neville Shone

Coping Successfully with Shyness
Margaret Oakes, Professor Robert Bor
and Dr Carina Eriksen

Coping with Anaemia
Dr Tom Smith

Coping with Drug Problems in the Family
Lucy Jolin

Coping with Early-onset Dementia
Jill Eckersley

Coping with Eating Disorders and Body Image
Christine Craggs-Hinton

Coping with Epilepsy
Dr Pamela Crawford and Fiona Marshall

Coping with Gout
Christine Craggs-Hinton

Coping with Guilt
Dr Windy Dryden

Coping with Liver Disease
Mark Greener

**Coping with Manipulation: When others
blame you for their feelings**
Dr Windy Dryden

Coping with Obsessive Compulsive Disorder
Professor Kevin Gournay, Rachel Piper
and Professor Paul Rogers

Depressive Illness – the Curse of the Strong
Dr Tim Cantopher

The Diabetes Healing Diet
Mark Greener and Christine Craggs-Hinton

Dying for a Drink
Dr Tim Cantopher

**The Empathy Trap: Understanding Antisocial
Personalities**
Dr Jane McGregor and Tim McGregor

**Epilepsy: Complementary and alternative
treatments**
Dr Sallie Baxendale

Fibromyalgia: Your Treatment Guide
Christine Craggs-Hinton

Hay Fever: How to beat it
Dr Paul Carson

The Heart Attack Survival Guide
Mark Greener

How to Beat Worry and Stress
Dr David Delvin

How to Come Out of Your Comfort Zone
Dr Windy Dryden

How to Eat Well When You Have Cancer
Jane Freeman

Living with Complicated Grief
Professor Craig A. White

Living with IBS
Nuno Ferreira and David T. Gillanders

Losing a Parent
Fiona Marshall

**Making Sense of Trauma: How to tell
your story**
Dr Nigel C. Hunt and Dr Sue McHale

Motor Neurone Disease: A family affair
Dr David Oliver

Natural Treatments for Arthritis
Christine Craggs-Hinton

Overcoming Loneliness
Alice Muir

The Panic Workbook
Dr Carina Eriksen, Professor Robert Bor
and Margaret Oakes

**Physical Intelligence: How to take charge
of your weight**
Dr Tom Smith

Reducing Your Risk of Dementia
Dr Tom Smith

**The Self-Esteem Journal: Using a journal
to build self-esteem**
Alison Waines

**Transforming Eight Deadly Emotions
into Healthy Ones**
Dr Windy Dryden

Treating Arthritis: The drug-free way
Margaret Hills and Christine Horner

Treating Arthritis: The supplements guide
Julia Davies

**When Someone You Love Has Depression:
A handbook for family and friends**
Barbara Baker

Overcoming Common Problems

The Empathy Trap: Understanding Antisocial Personalities

DR JANE McGREGOR
and
TIM McGREGOR

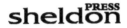

We dedicate this book to our son, Fin

First published in Great Britain in 2013

Sheldon Press
36 Causton Street
London SW1P 4ST
www.sheldonpress.co.uk

British Library Cataloguing-in-Publication Data
A catalogue record for this book is available from the British Library

ISBN 978–1–84709–276–2
eBook ISBN 978–1–84709–277–9

Typeset by Fakenham Prepress Solutions, Fakenham, Norfolk NR21 8NN
First printed in Great Britain by Ashford Colour Press
Subsequently digitally printed in Great Britain

eBook by Fakenham Prepress Solutions, Fakenham, Norfolk NR21 8NN

Produced on paper from sustainable forests

Contents

Acknowledgements

Without the many people who have shared their experiences of it openly and freely, the problem of sociopathic abuse might still remain hidden, so we give thanks to all those who helped in the creation of this book. Special thanks for their personal contributions go to Nancy Ellen Iandoli and Colleen Fourie, and also to Debrieanna, Paul and those individuals who contributed but prefer to remain anonymous. We owe Nancy a further debt of gratitude for her comments on early drafts of the book, as we do Fiona Marshall, commissioning editor at Sheldon Press, for her suggestions and encouragement.

Thanks also to Alison Gunson, founder of the Facebook group Children of Narcissistic Sociopathic Parents Support Group, and to its members, whose insights have greatly enriched the book. And we thank Simon Baron-Cohen, author of *Zero Degrees of Empathy*, for generously giving permission to reproduce his EQ (Empathy Quotient) test at the back of the book.

Lastly, we would like to thank all the super-empaths out there, past and present, for showing us the possibilities of the human spirit.

1

Introduction: what the book is about

This book is designed to heighten awareness of the problems of sociopathic abuse – and equip you to spot, avoid or remove sociopaths from your life.

Sociopaths are individuals with little or no conscience or ability to empathize with others' feelings. One sociopath (some people prefer the term psychopath) in the course of his or her lifetime will affect many, many people in a myriad harmful ways: bullying work colleagues, abusing children, instigating domestic violence or traumatizing friends and family through a sustained campaign of emotional abuse. Our purposes in writing the book are to reach out and offer supportive guidance to those who already have been targeted by a sociopath, and to forewarn and forearm others who want to reduce the likelihood of being a target of abuse themselves.

The book is also about harnessing your powers of empathy. On the one hand, empathic people prove eye-catching quarry to the sociopath; on the other, if the expression of empathy was more widely approved by society at large it could provide a powerful antidote to sociopathic abuse. This is the 'empathy trap' of the book's title.

Sociopaths in society

For simplicity's sake we use sociopath in the book as a catch-all term. Because the medical profession continues to debate the exact features of this condition, we will not be exploring it in detail. Our aim is to highlight not the condition itself, but the destructive effects of sharing your life with someone who has a sociopathic disorder.

Sociopaths are chameleon-like and lurk freely among us. They pose a serious threat to humankind, harming individuals, families and communities the world over, affecting the health and well-being of millions daily. Yet, for reasons explored in this book, they exist largely unseen; and this lack of awareness and responsiveness means that the traumas they inflict upon their many targets go undetected.

Sociopaths exist in greater numbers than you might suppose, although it is hard to know for sure just how many there are. Since most estimates are derived from data based on specific sub-groups like prison populations rather than the general population, and the condition has been subject to regular redefinition, estimates for sociopathy in society vary considerably. Martha Stout, a psychologist who treats the survivors of psychological trauma, informs us in her valuable book *The Sociopath Next Door* that 4 per cent of the general population are sociopathic. This estimate is derived from a large clinical trial involving primary care patients in the United States, which found that 8 per cent of men and 3.1 per cent of women met the criteria for a diagnosis of anti-social personality disorder (AsPD), one of the terms used to describe those displaying sociopathic traits. The frequency of the condition was higher (13.4 per cent for men and 4 per cent for women) for those people with a history of childhood conduct disorder (a precursor of adult sociopathy).[1] Meanwhile researchers Paul Babiak and Robert Hare estimate that 1 per cent of the population have the condition, with another 10 per cent or more falling into what they call the 'grey zone'. In their book *Snakes in Suits*,[2] Babiak and Hare suggest that the prevalence is likely to be higher in some groups including the business world, the philosophy and practices of which encourage sociopathic traits such as callousness and grasping behaviour.

Australian psychologist John Clarke has been working along the same lines as Babiak and Hare. In his book *Working with Monsters*[3] he reports that up to 0.5 per cent of women and 2 per cent of men could be classified as sociopathic (like Babiak and Hare he prefers the term 'psychopath'). A British study has estimated the prevalence of sociopathy in the general population at just under 1 per cent (approximately 620,000 people in the UK), although like other studies, this study found that prevalence is higher among certain groups including prisoners, the homeless, and people who have been admitted to psychiatric institutions.[4]

As you can see, estimates of sociopathy in the general population vary from less than 1 person in 100 to 1 in 25. Even at the more conservative end of the estimates, this translates into a possible 3.13 million sociopaths in the USA. And worldwide it equates to a figure of around 70 million. So the fact that sociopathic abuse remains such an overlooked problem is surprising, if not shocking.

The cruelty of sociopaths finds no bounds, for there is no recourse, treatment or punishment to permanently stop them.

Sociopath-induced distress and trauma

Individuals who have been targeted by a sociopath often respond with self-deprecating statements like 'I was stupid', 'What was I thinking?' or 'I should've listened to my gut instinct.' But being involved with a sociopath is like being brainwashed. The sociopath's superficial charm is usually the means by which he or she conditions people. On initial contact a sociopath will often test other people's empathy, so questions geared towards discovering whether you are highly empathetic or not should ring alarm bells. Those with a highly empathetic disposition are often targeted. Those who have lower levels of empathy are often passed over, though they may be drawn in and used by sociopaths as part of their cruel entertainment, as we discuss later in the book.

Those living with a sociopath usually exist in a state of constant emotional chaos. They may feel anxious and afraid, not knowing when the sociopath will fly into a rage. The sociopath meanwhile carries on untouched, using aggression, violence or emotional bullying to abuse his or her partner. Sociopaths are often aggressive, though not all of them exhibit violent or criminal behaviour. Aggression is not limited to men either; sociopathic women can be aggressive and violent too. Sociopaths make up 25 per cent of the prison population, committing more than twice as many violent and aggressive acts as other criminals do. Violent sociopaths who cheat on their partners or defraud people are the ones most likely to get caught. According to Robert Hare, the author of *Without Conscience*, in the United States approximately 20 per cent of male and female prisoners are sociopaths. They commit more than twice as many violent and aggressive acts as do other criminals and are responsible for more than 50 per cent of all serious crimes. When they get out of prison, they often return to crime. The reoffending rate of sociopaths is about double that of other offenders and for violent crimes it is triple.[5]

As well as inflicting physical trauma on others, there is the added and less visible burden of sociopath-induced emotional trauma, which if left unchecked can lead to anxiety disorders, depression and post-traumatic stress disorder (PTSD). Chronically traumatized people often exhibit hyper-vigilant, anxious and agitated behaviour. They may also experience insomnia and assorted somatic (bodily) symptoms such as tension headaches, gastrointestinal disturbances, abdominal pain, back pain, tremors and nausea. Exposure to and interaction with a sociopath in childhood can leave lifelong scars, including a deep mistrust of other people and anxiety in social situations. Yet for all these problems, no one knows the true extent or depth of mental anguish suffered by those on the receiving end of chronic sociopathic abuse, because in the majority of cases the physical and mental health problems either go undetected or the root cause is overlooked.

We believe that sociopathic abuse thus has a substantial public health dimension and as such warrants far more attention than it attracts at present. The public need to be more alert and equipped to counter the problem and to stop sociopaths from interfering in adverse ways in other people's lives. Furthermore, effective responses and interventions are required to reduce the range and extent of sociopathic abuse suffered by people the world over.

Defining the problem

As we stated at the outset, this book is not about sociopaths or the condition per se; it is about surviving the harm they cause. We will only set out to define the condition loosely, because we aren't convinced that current terminology and labels are especially useful. The distinctions between labels like sociopathy, anti-social personality disorder, borderline personality disorder (BPD), narcissistic personality disorder (NPD),[6] and psychopathy are blurred and confusing. In fact we hope at some point that psychiatry will get away entirely from the existing labels and redefine them all as conditions of low or zero empathy – something we discuss further over the next few pages. Nevertheless we feel some discussion of the changing conceptualization of sociopathy is justified, so we'll next highlight some key turning points in defining the problem.

The idea that there are people who look human but are not, and who exist without empathy or concern for the rest of humanity, was first mooted in 1801 by the physician Philippe Pinel (1745–1826).[7]

In his work *A Treatise on Insanity*, Pinel named the condition *manie sans délire*, which roughly translated means 'madness without delusion'. Some time later, an English doctor, J. C. Pritchard (1786–1848), ascribed the term 'moral insanity' to the condition. Pritchard described it as 'a form of mental derangement in which the intellectual faculties [are uninjured] while the disorder is manifested principally or alone in the state of feelings, temper or habits . . . The moral principles of the mind . . . are depraved or perverted, the power of self-government is lost or greatly impaired, and the individual is . . . incapable of conducting himself with decency and propriety in the business of life'.[8]

Nearly 100 years on, in 1941, American psychiatrist Hervey Cleckley published *The Mask of Sanity*, a book which first described the diagnostic criteria for the 'psychopathic personality'. This was based primarily on experience with adult male psychopaths hospitalized in a closed institution. From his observations Cleckley drew up a set of diagnostic criteria, including superficial charm, a lack of anxiety or guilt, undependability or dishonesty, egocentricity, an inability to form lasting intimate relationships, a failure to learn from punishment, poverty of emotions, a lack of insight into the impact of one's behaviour, and a failure to plan ahead. Interestingly his definition of a psychopath made no reference to physical aggression or breaking the law.

From our perspective, Cleckley's best definition of psychopathy comes in a later edition of the book, in which he described a psychopath as 'a biologic organism outwardly intact, showing excellent peripheral function, but centrally deficient or disabled'. We like both the elegance of this description and the way it pinpoints how hard it is to spot sociopaths given their ordinary outward appearance.

Subsequent to Cleckley's book, revisions of the classification were made by the American Psychiatric Association (APA). The classification of psychopathic personality was changed to that of sociopathic personality in 1958. In 1968 it was changed again to anti-social personality. After this Robert Hare elaborated on Cleckley's work to create the Psychopathy Checklist (PCL) and later a revised version, the PCL-R, which became the 'gold standard' assessment measure used to diagnose psychopathy. The PCL-R, which remains the standard measure today, identifies as typical of the psychopath interpersonal deficits such as grandiosity, arrogance and deceitfulness, affective deficits (lack of guilt and empathy), and impulsive and criminal behaviours.

Hare stated that the difference between psychopathy and sociopathy 'reflects the user's views on the origins and determinates of the clinical syndrome or disorder'. In other words some experts are convinced that the condition is forged entirely by social forces and call the condition **sociopathy**, whereas others are convinced that it is derived from a combination of psychological, biological and genetic factors and hence prefer the term **psychopathy**.[9]

Debate surrounding sociopathy and psychopathy and whether they are the same or different continues unabated today. The International Classification of Diseases diagnostic criteria of the World Health Organization (ICD-10) do not include psychopathy as a personality disorder and neither psychopathy nor sociopathy is currently referred to in diagnostic manuals, though both terms are widely used by mental health professionals and the public alike. In medical circles in recent years both terms have been replaced by the term anti-social personality disorder, though controversy over the definition of the disorder continues in debates over the American Psychiatric Association's upcoming Diagnostic and Statistical Manual of Mental Disorders V (DSM V). The current manual – DSM IV – puts emphasis on AsPD, but the criterion for AsPD lacks some key elements of sociopathy and psychopathy, with some experts regarding the current definition as describing criminality rather than sociopathy. Plenty more people can be diagnosed with AsPD than sociopathy or psychopathy, leaving the condition closer to the parameters of 'normal' human behaviour. In contrast the terms sociopathy and psychopathy help maintain the idea that the condition is distinct and extreme, hence serving to reassure the rest of us that the problem exists only in small numbers and only at the margins of society.

Adding to the debate, some theorists speculate that people behave cruelly not because they are intrinsically evil (a concept many consider outmoded), but because they lack empathy. According to Simon Baron-Cohen, an expert in developmental psychopathology at the University of Cambridge, limited or zero empathy may result from physical and psychological characteristics but empathy deficits can be turned around if people are taught to be more empathic. He points to the need to identify treatments (as yet none are available but trials are currently being conducted with families of children with conduct disorder, a child version of sociopathy) that will teach empathy to those who lack it.

Putting empathy under the microscope – or rather the modern-day gadgetry of functional magnetic resonance imaging (fMRI) – Baron-Cohen explores new ideas about empathy in his book *Zero Degrees of Empathy*.[10] He suggests that the level of empathy most of us experience varies according to the conditions we face at any given moment, although all of us have a predetermined level of empathy which we generally return to (our pre-set position, if you like) on what he calls the **empathy spectrum**. This spectrum ranges from six degrees at one end, down to zero degrees at the other. At six degrees we have highly empathic people, while at zero degrees we have the sociopath. For his research Baron-Cohen constructed an Empathy Quotient or EQ test that is intended as a measure to determine how easily you pick up on and how strongly you are affected by others' feelings. This is accessible online and we have also included it at the back of this book (see the Appendix).

Baron-Cohen also suggests that deep in the brain lies the **empathy circuit**. This is thought to involve at least ten interconnected brain regions, all regions of what is termed the 'social brain'. The first is the medial prefrontal cortex (MPFC), which is thought of as the 'hub' for social information processing and considered important for comparing your own perspective to someone else's. The functioning of this circuit determines where we each lie on the empathy spectrum, Baron-Cohen suggests. This idea relates to the earlier work of Giacomo Rizzolatti, a renowned Italian neurophysiologist. Rizzolatti demonstrated the existence of a system of nerve cells which he called **mirror neurons**. His work with primates showed that these nerve cells were fired not only when the animal performed an action, but when it saw another animal performing the same action. This suggests that empathy involves some form of mirroring of other people's actions and emotions. Using fMRI, scientists have identified which regions of the brain appear to be involved in the mirror neuron system.[11]

Scientists have been quick to equate mirror neurons with empathy, but this may be pushing the idea too far. We are still some way from understanding exactly how social and biological determinants interact. Besides, mirror neurons may just be the building blocks for empathy. Other mechanisms may be involved and be just as, if not more, significant. For instance, one region of the brain, the amygdala, is considered to be important in the empathy circuit (in fact we have two amygdalae in our brains, one in each hemisphere). The amygdalae appear to play a key role in emotional learning and regulation processing, and are vital in cueing us to look at other people's eyes when we want clues about their thoughts and emotions.

Outline of the book

This book alerts you to the ruses and manipulations sociopaths use and shows you how to invest in your empathic powers to keep them at bay. In Chapter 2 we introduce the tell-tale signs of sociopathy and sociopathic abuse by providing accounts drawn from real-life situations. In Chapter 3, 'A profile of the sociopath', we scrutinize the character of the sociopath in order to help you 'see' the problem behaviour for what it is. We hope that by reading the narratives and information about sociopaths' common traits you will begin to understand the characteristics of the sociopath and sociopathic behaviour.

In Chapter 4, 'Interactions of the sociopath', we analyse sociopaths' relations with other people, and in particular draw the reader's attention to the existence of what we call the Sociopath-Empath-Apath Triad (SEAT for short). This is important to appreciate because sociopaths' interactions frequently involve not only the chosen target (often a person with a high level of empathy) but an apathetic third party that we refer to as an 'apath'. How these three players interact is discussed in detail, as is the unfortunate reality that sociopaths frequently enlist the help of apaths in their cruel sport.

Chapter 5, 'Coping in the aftermath of a destructive relationship', is about the early days following sociopathic trauma. In this chapter we include things to watch out for and ways to cope in the immediate aftermath of an association, friendship or intimate relationship with a sociopath.

In Chapter 6, 'Establishing boundaries and regaining control of your life', we focus on the process of recovery and look at measures to help you get life back on track, while in Chapter 7 we discuss dealing with complex family situations. In Chapter 8 we explore the potential for long-term recovery from sociopathic trauma, and in the final sections of the book, 'Useful addresses' and 'Further reading and resources', we list useful books, online resources and other forms of information and support.

2

Everyday sociopaths

How do sociopaths work, and how can you spot them in everyday life? The purpose of this chapter is to heighten your awareness of the nature of sociopaths. Many sociopaths wreak havoc in a covert way, so that their underlying condition remains hidden for years. They may possess a superficial charm, and this appeal diverts attention from the more disturbing aspects of their nature.

Another reason that their real natures remain hidden is that many of the behaviours exhibited by sociopaths are seen in ordinary people too. Quite a lot of people cheat on their partners, have addiction problems, steal and lie, but not everybody who does so is sociopathic. Nevertheless sociopaths are more numerous than is generally supposed and we encounter them on a daily basis, even if we don't register the fact. They may be your neighbour, your partner, your boss, or the person next to you in the checkout queue. So it is quite probable that if you don't know one intimately, you have fleeting contact with a few.

Case histories

The following accounts of sociopathic behaviour are drawn from real-life situations. Though they do not constitute an exhaustive account of everyday sociopaths or encounters, they reflect the kind of sociopathic behaviour and abuse that goes on in the course of everyday life.

As we've said, sociopaths come in all shapes and forms – men, women and even children – and can be hard to spot. We hope the following case histories illustrate just how individuals may be systematically targeted until they feel they can barely trust their own sense of reality – what we call 'gaslighting' (see Chapter 4). Sociopathic abuse is targeted abuse. Sadly, it can wreck lives, though we also hope to show that victims can become survivors, even if at huge cost.

The sociopathic spouse

Susan, 47, was a teacher. With menopause looming, she realized that it wouldn't be too long before retirement was on the horizon, and she was beginning to be restless. A placid, kindly woman, she had been escaping daily to her little primary school as a way of getting away from home, where her husband Peter ruled. He was a retired teacher who still did supply work, but was spending increasing amounts of time at home. Once she'd cooked him breakfast and he'd approved her clothes for the day, she was free to go – her salary, paid of course into their joint account, was a welcome supplement to his income. (He profoundly disapproved of her maintaining her own bank account, in which she was only allowed to keep a token amount.) Peter didn't want to hear too much about her day when she returned, when he was often moody or sulky – or off on his own hobby of golf – but again she was more than welcome to cook supper later on when he was ready for it.

Control, and being in control, is of key importance to sociopaths. Peter was never physically violent, but he would erode Susan's self-confidence with constant criticisms – of her weight, clothes, appearance and achievements in general. 'I was always being measured and assessed, and usually just not doing well enough – it was like living with the head teacher who was always marking you,' she said. He would try and control which friends she saw – in fact, he preferred her not to see any. Likewise, he had tried to cut her off from her family early in their married life, saying that her parents had personality disorders and her sisters were fools. Indeed, he displayed another typical sociopathic trait – he was hyper-critical; no one was ever good enough, and as a couple they were socially isolated. In spite of this, Susan's naturally sociable nature won the day and she managed to have friends and a social circle away from home, which stood her in good stead later.

In many ways, though, it was a lonely life, especially as Peter was also physically distant – what intimacy there had been between them had long since dwindled. If ever Susan tried to rock the boat, Peter became threatening and aggressive. Susan loved the children at the school dearly, but it wasn't enough. She did something entirely out of character and had a brief liaison with Stephen, a social worker who was supporting one of the pupils. The affair, coming so late in the day, was a last-ditch cry for help. She was not much good at cheating so it ended no sooner than it began and she confessed everything to Peter.

Peter said little at first, but over the next few days he took his revenge; he told their three children. He managed to make a shocking story of it and, although they were adult and lived away from home, they felt the bond of trust had been destroyed, and that their mother had behaved abominably. He told them that Susan had neglected them as children, that she was an alcoholic, and that she had behaved erratically and cruelly towards him. Being highly articulate and forceful, Peter talked the children down if they ventured to doubt the stories, and said that Susan had done a good job of deceiving them.

Susan was devastated. For 25 years her life had revolved around her family's wants and needs and, in particular, around Peter. She felt her life was over, and that none of her children would ever trust her again. Then, Peter suddenly announced that he was leaving, and said he would fight Susan tooth and nail for the house and money.

In fact, he didn't have a leg to stand on – Susan got a good solicitor and managed to secure her rightful share of their possessions. While sorting through papers prior to the move, she came across some which made it plain that Peter had had several affairs. Susan hadn't known that Peter had his own circle and inner coterie – another common hallmark of sociopaths is secrecy and a double life, and Peter's 'golf', as well as comprising many cronies whom Susan never met, also included a mistress of many years' standing as well as more casual liaisons.

Susan felt she was well rid of her sociopathic spouse, and only wondered that she'd put up with it for so long. Her life took a lot of rebuilding, but she had several long-standing friendships she'd made at the school, both with other teachers and with parents, and she was a well-known and well-loved member of the community. Once the break with Peter was made, she was surprised at how many people offered support and came out against Peter – one of them, Gerry, even offered to marry her.

As she felt she needed some time on her own, Susan refused, but said she'd reconsider in two years' time if he was still willing. Meanwhile they're building a long-term friendship based on mutual respect, while Susan comes to terms with the aftermath of her relationship with Peter, with the help of a counsellor. She is also rebuilding her relationship with her children – and trying to get them used to the fact that she is no longer the doormat she might have been when they were growing up.

The sociopathic parent – Rebecca's story

Motherhood did not come naturally to my mother. It took me several years to realize that she genuinely didn't feel any real affection for me as a baby – she felt trapped, tied down, and hated most aspects of caring. This might happen to any new mother, but in our case there was much more to it. She never got used to parenthood, which she referred to as 'the life sentence' – I think she always regarded me as a nuisance and it took me a long time to realize that she disliked me just for being what I was. She was cold and distant, with fits of vindictive rage in which she would beat me and lock me in a cupboard under the stairs; once, she hacked off chunks of my hair. She repeatedly told me I was worthless and with time I came to believe it. To divert attention from the abuse, she ensured that I was always well dressed – though few people got to see us out and about together. As another distracting device, she developed an extreme case of agoraphobia and other psychosomatic (I now think) disorders, took antidepressants by the bucketful and spent a lot of time in bed. We were quite isolated from the world and I assumed that this was how it had to be.

My father adored me, and I adored him. He could not help, however. He was a mild, kind man, not very ambitious, and my mother had only agreed to marry him if he provided her with the very best. As he loved her dearly, he agreed and worked like a slave. While I was growing up, my mother grew to resent the attention my father gave me, and did all she could to keep us apart, but when he came home at night and showered me with hugs and kisses, I was as happy as anything. He was totally oblivious to Mum's resentment and to all the manifestations of the abuse, including all the injuries and bruises. I tried hard not to rock the boat, and said nothing, and the bruises were largely hidden behind my expensive clothes.

The abuse continued all through my childhood and had a corrosive effect. By the time I was in my late teens I was emotionally spent. What saved me from despair was my passion for learning. I left school with excellent grades and secured a place at a university, many miles from the family home, where I flourished, away from my mother's abuse.

At university I met and married Mike. Mike had had a troubled upbringing and came from a broken home. I believed this was a bond and that our shared understanding of life meant we were the perfect match. After university we both found good jobs, and everything seemed to be working out.

But I found marriage lonelier than I expected. Our perfect understanding didn't last – Mike took to drink and he became violent and aggressive towards me, even when I was pregnant (we had two children). There was the increasing distance between my father and me. My mother employed all manner of tactics to block contact – she intercepted mail, arranged long weekends away when I wanted to visit, and always answered the phone. Dad and I seldom spoke and eventually I thought he was rejecting me.

Over the next few years our problems escalated along with our debts after Mike lost his job through his drinking. I had no one to turn to, and had more or less lost touch with my parents. Then one day out of the blue my mother rang and said my father was ill, and that she needed my help paying the bills. I tried to explain we were deeply in debt ourselves but the call ended in a horrible row.

I never saw my father again. Six months later he died in hospital. My mother didn't even tell me until the next day. When she did call, it was to inform me that she'd persuaded Dad to write me out of his will.

Many sociopaths are women and, like others of their kind, appear to get away with it, leaving scars of various sorts in their wake. Perhaps the only mitigating factor to be put forward is that they truly 'don't know what they're missing'. Rebecca's mother never saw her grandchildren (and indeed Rebecca was keen to protect them from the possible effects of further abuse). There seemed to be a whole dimension of life to which Rebecca's mother was, as it were, colour-blind. With time, Rebecca was able to struggle through to this dimension and to see that life was a larger and kinder affair than she had found it as a child – though this took time and a great deal of counselling.

The sociopath at work

Mary had a narrow escape, although she didn't think so at the time. As office receptionist, she came in for the full blast of John's 'charm' – fulsome compliments about what a sterling job she did, and poor-me comments about how hard he worked, designed to evoke her sympathy. He gave her lifts home and talked with a sad face about how Clive, his boss, was against him and did everything to block his career. Widowed early in life, Mary had no plans to remarry and did not go out of her way to attract men, but, with John, she might have been tempted. Vistas of a new life opened before her – and once they had appeared, it was hard to ignore them. She began to dress more stylishly, to lose weight, and to have her hair coloured and permed.

Being bright and observant as well as lonely, however, she watched him with some attention. It all seemed a little too good to be true. She noted that he could drop the charm like a cloak when he wished, revealing a very definite, almost dogmatic manner beneath. She also noted how he flirted with Kylie, the office beauty (who, wisely, didn't respond to his advances) – and how often he looked at himself in the mirror. Mary also saw how John 'accidentally' took a chip out of his boss Clive's new car while parking one morning, and how he managed to get Kylie blamed for this as a 'woman driver'. He also spread a rumour that Kylie had been brought in by the central management team to close the office down. His tensions with his boss Clive escalated and John finally lodged a formal complaint of unprofessional conduct against him. Mary began to wonder. Magnetic as he was, John seemed to attract just a little too much trouble – though it was still lovely to be confided in and told how well she understood.

John's comeuppance reached him from an unexpected direction – the RSPCA. Neighbours had notified them that he treated his young Labrador badly, keeping her locked up in the garage all day with inadequate water and food – indeed he only kept the dog to hurt his ex-wife, who adored it. All this came to Mary's ears via a neighbour and when she asked John about it, the mask slipped. He stuttered out some excuse about the dog being ill, but Mary had seen through him.

For Mary, the positive effect of coming into contact with John was feeling that she could perhaps be attractive to men again after losing her husband. On the negative side though, her confidence was severely dented. She doubted her ability to make wise choices in relationships, and felt she had been a 'mug' to be so deliberately used in one of John's complicated games. Like Susan, Mary felt she was well rid of this 'charmer' in her life – but she should have seen through him earlier, she felt. Her hurt lasted for quite some time.

The school bully

James, 15, was an only child, privileged, bright and supremely confident. Despite his undoubted advantages, however, he was often bored and listless, skiving off school with faked illnesses and finding it easy to manipulate his parents.

At school James took a dislike to a classmate, Sam, who was sensitive and popular. He would mock him for auditioning for a part in the school play, or for getting upset over failing a geography test. The situation deteriorated when it became known that Sam's parents were separating. Sam appeared to be taking it all with fortitude, to the admiration of his peers. Sam also got attention and sympathy from the school staff, especially from James's 'favourite' teacher – or the teacher he found it easiest to manipulate.

James decided on a master plan of covert bullying. Using the class gossip, he started a whispering campaign implying that Sam's parents weren't splitting up, and that he had only said they were in order to seek attention. Sadly, this was all too successful and over the next few days Sam was met with silence and verbal bullying from his hitherto supportive classmates, a situation which escalated into a physical fight in which Sam was knocked out.

Unbelievably, James continued his campaign, targeting several of Sam's close friends over the next few days. They found themselves accused of quite serious misdemeanours – stealing money, and sending offensive emails and insulting text messages. Finally, just as things began to settle down, the 'favourite' teacher went on 'leave with immediate effect' after accusations of physical assault and violence towards a pupil. Where had the accusations come from? James knew.

While it seems hard to believe that one young schoolboy could cause such havoc, this case history demonstrates how deliberately sociopaths can and do target others. Taking advantage of people's general credibility and good will, and of the school structure and culture, James exploited the situation with almost uncanny insight and destructive flair. With a more perceptive head teacher, James might perhaps have been found out, but like so many sociopaths he knew just whom to manipulate and just how far he could go. He has since left the school, his parents claiming he 'wasn't understood' there, and continues his activities in a new school.

In the next chapter we'll explore the characteristic behaviours of everyday sociopaths like the ones described here.

3

A profile of the sociopath

To deal with sociopaths effectively you first need to open your eyes – which is why, in this chapter, we'll be putting the sociopath under the microscope. In the tale 'The Emperor's New Clothes' by Hans Christian Andersen, two weavers promise the Emperor a new suit of clothes that is invisible to those who are stupid and unfit for their positions. When the Emperor parades before his subjects all the adults, not wishing to be seen in a negative light, pretend they see the Emperor's elegant new clothes. The only truthful person in the crowd is a child, who cries out, 'But he isn't wearing any clothes!'

In this chapter we'll help you see sociopaths in the same way the boy in the tale sees the Emperor – naked, and as they really are. Very young children often have this ability – they'll say things like 'That's unkind, stop it', or 'I'm telling on you, you bully', when they see behaviour that defies the social boundaries that they have been taught.

But as children get older, most find it gets harder to take such a bold stance. From infancy we are trained to 'toe the line', to conform to society's standards and rules. We are conditioned to keep quiet, which often means turning a blind eye or putting up with abuse. The boy in the tale represents those who see the problem behaviour for what it is and find the courage of their convictions to make a stand. 'Sight' becomes insight, which turns into action. Awareness is the first step in limiting the negative effects of contact with a sociopath.

Traits of the sociopath

Superficial charm

Have you ever come across someone with magnetic charm? Perhaps alongside this he affects an air of importance and has a grandiose view of himself? Sociopathic charm is not like any other. It is not in the least self-conscious. Sociopaths rarely exhibit social inhibitions, so they hardly ever get anxious or tongue-tied. Nor are they afraid of offending you. They aren't held back by the social convention that ensures most of us take turns in talking. They talk *at* you, confident that you will agree with everything they say.

Often they have a lot to say. A 'conversation' with a sociopath can feel like a bombardment. To the untrained ear sociopaths' pronouncements sound authoritative because they tend to use words and phrases intended to make them sound knowledgeable, but which on dissection sometimes prove nothing more than gobbledygook. This peculiarity in their mode of expression can be exacerbated by their use of muddled-up phrases and mixed metaphors. No one really knows why this is the case, but it seems to be a common feature.

When you first meet a sociopath, you may be impressed by her good manners. She tends to be charming at first, may go out of her way to please you and often falls back on flattery. These tactics are designed to draw you in. But beware, for she is not what she appears, which is why sociopaths are often called 'social chameleons'. It seems counterintuitive that someone so charming can be so dangerous, but many people are duped this way. Being charming is a sociopath's most potent trait. Targets often later remark that they were overwhelmed by the sociopath's charm offensive. He may seem larger than life, a go-getter, an adventurer. His grandiose air and smooth conversation add to the illusion of being in the presence of someone special. He makes you feel boring and insipid by comparison.

Everything a sociopath does is calculated to have an effect on you. Just as his charm is superficial, so too is everything else about him. The smile *looks* phoney because it *is* phoney. The sociopath has blunt emotional reactions and fakes emotions to appear sincere. Occasionally you might catch him looking closely at your mouth as you speak, as though mouthing words and rehearsing. One commonly observed habit is frequent pursing of the lips or chewing the sides of the mouth, while he may twist and contort his mouth in peculiar ways. It is not clear why sociopaths do any of these things. Perhaps they are practising facial expressions, or perhaps there is some physical reason. But the only natural smile you will see exhibited by a sociopath is a sneer as he derives pleasure from seeing others suffer.

It is hard to recognize the shameless. In her book *The Sociopath Next Door*, Martha Stout claims that the sociopath will make it his business to know how a person can be manipulated, hence his use of flattery and charm. It is quite common for sociopaths to create a sense of similarity and intimacy. They will tell you that only you understand them, that you are their special 'soul mate'. In our earlier case histories all the central characters possessed this quality in varying degrees. John the workplace bully is a master of flattery. He compliments Mary in order to 'play' her and to unwittingly involve her in his sociopathic games. Our 15-year-old schoolboy James possesses a phoney charm. He uses it to blindside those in authority. As a consequence, no one guesses he is manipulating everyone behind the scenes. In other sociopaths, such as Peter, the 'charm offensive' is more muted.

The need for stimulation

Another characteristic of sociopaths is their need for constant stimulation. They become bored easily, perhaps because their emotional repertoire is so limited. Their heads are not full of the kind of emotions that distract the rest of us. It is hard to imagine what life must be like without constant emotional 'noise'. The rest of us have it, though we are not always aware of the fact. Occasionally this emotional noise comes to the fore; maybe when we're stressed or anxious over an exam or an illness or when experiencing bereavement, when we are far more aware of the commotion whirring around inside.

Sociopaths, on the other hand, have a very limited emotional range and are noted for their shallowness and fleeting attachments. Consequently they don't get other people's 'neediness' and see no point in showing emotions or sharing feelings except as an act of manipulation. Instead, and to fill the void, they tend to seek stimulation from external sources. They engage in 'mind games' (a struggle for psychological one-upmanship), and employ behaviour to specifically demoralize or empower their target. In this way they undermine their targets' confidence in their own perceptions. The sociopath may invalidate other people's experience: not only its significance and content but the person's capacity to trust her recollection of events, hence making the person feel guilty for holding her original view. Such abusive mind games may include discounting (denial of the person's reality), diverting, trivializing, undermining, threatening and anger.

The sociopath's need for stimulation is illustrated in our case history involving James, the schoolboy who often gets bored and plays mind games on others to relieve his boredom. John, the workplace sociopath, is in constant need of stimulation too and hurts others simply for the kick of it. He also has a strong competitive streak, another feature of the sociopath.

Not all competitive people are sociopathic, clearly. What we are talking about here is aggressive behaviour where the sociopath misuses others in order to beat off rivals and pushes ahead regardless of whether others get hurt or not. Because they are indifferent to others, sociopaths do not display a proper sense of social responsibility. They develop strategies which allow them to ignore social convention, reason and evidence in the pursuit of some personal goal. Sociopaths may well believe they exhibit extraordinary social responsibility, and unfortunately society often colludes in this.

A parasitic lifestyle

Another commonly observed characteristic of the sociopath is a parasitic nature. To someone targeted by a sociopath with strong parasitic tendencies it can feel quite literally as if life is being sucked out of them. Parasitic behaviour is associated with passive aggression.[1] Passive aggressives do not deal with things directly. They talk behind your back and put others in the position of telling you what they would not say themselves. They find subtle ways of letting you know they are not happy. They are unlikely to show their angry or resentful nature. They conceal it behind a façade of affability, politeness, and a show of well-meaning. However, underneath there is usually manipulation going on.

Types of passive aggression include **victimization** – a situation where the person concerned is unable to look at his own part in a situation and turns the tables to become the victim, or at least to behave like one; **self-pity** – the 'poor me' scenario; **blaming** others for situations rather than being able to take responsibility for one's own actions; **withholding** usual behaviours or roles in order to reinforce to the other party that you are angry; and **learned helplessness**, where a person acts as if he cannot help himself. It is common for someone acting in this way to deliberately do a poor job of something to make a point. The important thing to note is that passive aggression is a destructive pattern of behaviour and a form of emotional abuse. Such behaviours cause great distress to the target, who often feels overburdened with guilt and responsibility.[2]

Manipulative behaviour

Psychological manipulation is a mainstay of the sociopath, who uses behaviour to influence or control others in a deceptive and dishonest way. Advancing the interests of the manipulator, often at another's expense, such methods are exploitative, abusive, devious and deceptive.

Manipulators may control their victims through **positive reinforcement**, which involves employing praise, superficial charm, superficial sympathy (crocodile tears) and excessive apologies, money, approval and gifts, attention, and the use of facial expressions such as a forced laughter or smiles, all for public recognition. Another approach is **negative reinforcement** – removing the person from a negative situation as a reward; for example, 'You won't have to pay all those bills if you allow me to move in with you.' Yet other means are **intermittent or partial reinforcement**, used to create a climate of fear and doubt, and **punishment**, including nagging, intimidation, threats, swearing, emotional blackmail and crying as ways of playing the victim.

A sociopathic manipulator can cause you to believe you are going crazy. If you find yourself in a relationship where you think you need to keep a record of what's been said and begin to question your own sanity, likely as not you are experiencing emotional manipulation. A sociopath is an expert in turning things around, rationalizing, justifying and explaining things away. He lies so smoothly and argues so persuasively that you begin to doubt your own senses. Over a period of time this is so eroding it can distort your sense of reality. The sociopath can make you feel guilty for speaking up or not speaking out, for being emotional or not being emotional enough, for caring or for not caring enough. Manipulation is a powerful strategy. Most of us are conditioned to check ourselves, and we are usually our own worst critics. If accused of being in the wrong or acting imperfectly we do whatever is necessary to reduce our feelings of guilt.

Another powerful strategy is to demand sympathy from us. The sociopath plays the victim remarkably well. However he seldom fights his own fights or does his own dirty work. In our earlier case history James manipulates Sam's friends, first by encouraging a pupil to start a whispering campaign and then by feeding the hostilities that saw fellow pupils gang up and attack Sam. Manipulators also use verbal abuse, explosive anger or other intimidating behaviour to establish dominance or superiority; even one incident of such behaviour can condition or train the target to avoid upsetting, confronting or contradicting the manipulator.[3]

According to psychologists Babiak and Hare, sociopaths are always on the lookout for individuals to scam or swindle. They outline the sociopathic approach as having three phases.[4]

The assessment phase

Some sociopaths will take advantage of almost anyone they meet, while others are more patient, waiting for the perfect, innocent target to cross their path. In each case, the sociopath is sizing up the potential usefulness of an individual as a source of money, power or influence. Some sociopaths enjoy a challenge while others prey on people who are vulnerable. During the assessment phase, the sociopath determines a potential target's weak points and uses these to lead the target off course.

The manipulation phase

In this phase the sociopath has identified a target and the manipulation begins. At this time a sociopath may create a persona or mask, specifically designed to 'work' for his or her target.

A sociopath will lie to gain the trust of her target. Sociopaths' lack of empathy and guilt allows them to lie with impunity; they do not see the value of telling the truth unless it will help them get what they want. As the interaction with the target proceeds, the sociopath carefully assesses the target's persona. This move gives her a picture of the target's traits and characteristics so she can exploit them. The target's persona may also reveal insecurities or weaknesses he wishes to hide from view.

The sociopath will eventually build a personal relationship with the target based on this knowledge. The persona of the sociopath, the 'personality' the target is bonding with, does not really exist. It is built on lies, carefully woven together to entrap the targeted person. It is a mask, one of many, customized to fit the target's particular expectations. This act of manipulation is predatory in nature and often leads to severe physical or emotional harm for the person targeted. Healthy relationships are built on mutual respect and trust; the targeted person believes mistakenly that the 'bond' between himself and the sociopath is of that kind, and that this is the reason their relationship is so successful. So when the sociopath behaves disrespectfully or there are breaches of trust, such incidences are overlooked.

The abandonment phase

This is when the sociopath decides that his target is no longer useful. He then abandons his target and moves on to a new one. Sometimes, perhaps not surprisingly, targets overlap. The sociopath can have several individuals 'on the go' as it were: one who has just been abandoned, but who is kept in the picture just in case the others do not work out; another who is currently being played; and a third, who is being groomed in readiness.

Pathological lying

The fact is that sociopaths lie. There are two recognized categories of people who constantly lie: compulsive and pathological. The first – compulsive liars – lie out of habit. There is no real reason, and they normally don't lie intentionally to hurt anyone. The latter – pathological liars – lie for altogether different reasons. This category is the kind into which sociopaths usually fall. Sociopathic liars lie to gain something. Their lying is often calculated and cunning. Sociopaths don't care who their lies will affect, as long as the lie fits their purpose and achieves what they want. Unlike compulsive liars, sociopathic liars can help themselves. They may well know the difference between right and wrong, but the crux of the matter is they don't care – though they can be so good at lying that they believe their own lies.

Pathological lying is an invaluable tool for a sociopath, who uses it to gain pity and sympathy. If you pay very close attention you may catch a sociopath in a lie because she has a tendency to tell different versions of the same lie to different people. However, the sociopath is apt to make sure that individuals who have been told different stories don't have the chance to meet or compare stories. She may even keep friends and acquaintances apart to minimize the risk of being exposed. And even if she is exposed, the sociopath doesn't baulk at telling a new lie to cover the old. Always remember when dealing with a sociopath that lying doesn't worry her one jot. Your feelings don't matter. The sociopath doesn't have the capability or desire to care about you. Nobody is 'special' to a sociopath unless they're serving her a purpose.

Sociopaths are highly likely to lie about their credentials; for example, when applying for a job a sociopath might well fake his curriculum vitae. Don't be surprised if you find out that your sociopath boss never got a degree, let alone graduated from Cambridge, as stated in his CV! Sociopaths are also likely to lie about previous relationships. Teenage sociopaths are likely to lie about situational circumstances: James, our school bully, lied about the situation that Sam faced at home and was covert in his efforts to bring him down. He also had no qualms in making up accusations about his teacher being violent towards a pupil.

Sociopaths are equally likely to lie about physical or mental abuse, especially if it will help them in a divorce or custody situation. Pathological lying is persistent lying. It doesn't matter if the lies are easily disproved, because for some illogical reason they are seldom challenged. The lies sociopaths create may be fantastic in nature, extensive, elaborate and complicated. Often there is a blurring between fiction and reality. The magnitude of the lie or its callous nature is irrelevant, and so are any consequences. Such characteristics have led researchers to conclude that the lying behaviour might be gratifying in itself, and the expected reward external.[5]

Faking illness

A lot of sociopaths lie about being ill, or about being in recovery from serious illnesses. They behave in this way to gain attention or evoke your sympathy. No matter how bad your situation, the sociopath has experienced it ten times worse. A person adopting this type of behaviour exaggerates or creates symptoms of illness in order to gain attention, sympathy and comfort. It is a form of hypochondriasis, though it is unlikely that the sociopath actually believes he has a disease. It is common for sociopaths to feign serious illnesses: rare conditions, or life-threatening ones like cancer. By mimicking illness the sociopath may be seeking financial compensation or your undivided care and attention. Whatever his goal, the basis of it is to seek advantages and personal profit he would not otherwise get. This is probably the driving force behind James's frequent fake illnesses.

Feigning illness is also a habit of Rebecca's sociopathic mother. Her frequent illnesses and obsessive behaviours are tactics designed to gain attention and sympathy from her husband and get more control at home.

Aggression and anti-social behaviour

When a sociopath is sad or angry everyone knows it, for she can fly into terrible rages. Sociopaths exhibit anger or attempt to gain your pity when intent on deceiving you. They rely on the fact that your judgement will be affected by your conscience and feelings of guilt if you don't respond to the situation sensitively or fairly.

In our case studies there are many examples of anti-social behaviour and most are dressed up as something else by our expert manipulators. James, for example, is already a master of the clandestine, an expert covert aggressive. His ability to tell lies is matched by his convincing ability to feign outrage. His *pièce de résistance* is his allegation of physical assault against his supposed favourite teacher. These overt displays of emotion, while fake, often persuade the 'bit part' players to accept the sociopath's view of events.

Manipulation must occur for us not to 'see' the aggression and anti-social behaviour for what it is. The process obscures our view so that the sociopath can 'get away with murder'. This is how Rebecca's mother manages to get away with physically and emotionally tormenting her daughter while keeping her behaviour hidden from her husband. The sociopath's reliance on bullying and sabotage as an act of aggression frequently also reveals itself in the workplace. John, our workplace sociopath, is very competitive. Although frequent in sociopaths, this trait is in any case commonplace in society. The worlds of school and work in effect promote it, and nowhere is this more apparent than in commerce and politics.

In our story John is not just competitive; he is covertly aggressive to others. He shows vindictiveness to other human beings and extreme cruelty to his dog. Cruelty to animals is thought to be common among sociopaths. Nevertheless sociopaths are just as likely to use pets as a prop; as a way of convincing a new target of their kind-heartedness and trustworthiness.

Another aspect of sociopathic cruelty is child-on-child cruelty. A real-life case is the death of little Jamie Bulger, a toddler murdered by two ten-year-old boys in Liverpool in 1993. That two ten-year-olds could commit such a heinous crime was received with disbelief. So was the more recent case of 14-year-old Daniel Bartlam, who hit his mother seven times with a claw hammer at their home in Nottingham. These cases show that sociopathic children aren't too hard to find, even if the word 'sociopath' is never mentioned in the reporting of such cases. This state of being is so far removed from our understanding of what it is to be young and human, it seems, that we refuse to speak its name.

Lack of empathy and remorse

Simon Baron-Cohen, author of *Zero Degrees of Empathy*,[6] defines empathy as an ability to identify what someone else is thinking or feeling, and to respond to their thoughts and feelings with an appropriate emotion. What causes people to be capable of seriously hurting one another is not rightly understood, but when our empathy is 'switched off' and we operate solely on an 'I' basis (viewing the world as if only we existed), we are much more inclined to view other people as objects. This is the standpoint from which sociopaths are thought to see the rest of us.

Baron-Cohen suggests that we all stand somewhere on an empathy spectrum (from high to low) in a relatively stable position, though this is not immovable. In other words, you may experience quite a high level of empathy in general but your ability to empathize with others may display an occasional 'blip'. The good news is that for most of us our empathy is recoupable. For those with a long-standing lack of empathy, unfortunately it is not.

A side effect of having no empathy is that sociopaths take no responsibility for their own behaviour. It is always about what has been done to them. One of the easiest ways to spot a sociopath is that he often attempts to establish intimacy through the early sharing of deeply personal information that is generally intended to make you feel sorry for him. Initially you may perceive this type of person as very sensitive, emotionally open, even a little vulnerable. However, that couldn't be further from the truth. Sociopaths are addicted to high drama. Life with a sociopath always entails having to deal with numerous problems and crises.

But don't expect the sociopath in your life to feel sorry for anyone but himself. As we keep emphasizing, sociopaths are defined by their lack of empathy and remorse. It is apparent that James the schoolboy doesn't care one iota that he fabricated an allegation of assault by his teacher. He cared not one jot that he got this teacher into trouble with the education authorities or that the poor man was in danger of losing his job. He didn't care that Sam was struggling to cope with a family breakdown, or that Sam was beaten up by his peers because of his lies and actions. James cares for no one but himself; he probably doesn't feel love or affection for anyone, even his parents. Likewise, John our workplace sociopath doesn't feel the slightest guilt for tarnishing his boss's reputation with a complaint of professional misconduct.

Gender differences

There has been little systematic investigation of sociopathy in women. In fact previous research has been over-reliant both on a male conceptualization of the disorder and on means of assessment developed, and primarily validated, with men.[7] Furthermore, since sociopathy is not routinely assessed in women the harmful potential of some sociopathic women can be overlooked, especially towards their partners and children.

From the available literature it would seem that when women direct their aggression towards others, their victims are generally those within their domestic sphere of control – a partner, a family member, a child, a friend or a work colleague. In addition, much of the harm or aggression carried out by women involves manipulation of, or damage to, peer relationships through aggressive competitiveness, the withdrawal of friendship, ostracism, overt bullying, telling lies about the victim to promote her rejection by others and other acts of interpersonal aggression, in order to exclude the victim from the social group. Conversely, when men direct their aggression toward others, its function is to damage the victim's sense of control or dominance over the perpetrator of the aggression. Male aggression is more visible and more likely to result in arrest and punishment than is the case with women.[8]

In the next chapter we'll examine sociopaths' social interactions and how they use and abuse other people for their own sport.

4

Interactions of the sociopath

Instead of living for, in, and with yourself, as a reasonable being ought, you seek only to fasten your feebleness on some other person's strength.

(Charlotte Brontë, *Jane Eyre*, ch. 21)

In this chapter we analyse sociopathic social interactions. In particular we'll be drawing your attention to the existence of what we have termed the Sociopath-Empath-Apath Triad (SEAT). Unremitting abuse of other people is an activity of the sociopath that stands out above the rest. To win their games, sociopaths enlist the help of hangers-on, which means that their interactions frequently involve not only the chosen target but a third party we call the **apath** – we'll explain why below.

The apath

In the context of any sociopathic interaction we call those that collude in the sport of the sociopath **apathetic**, or 'apaths' for short. An apath is the type of person most likely to do the sociopath's bidding. Being apathetic in this situation means showing a lack of concern or being indifferent to the targeted person. In Chapter 3 we highlighted the importance of 'seeing' the problem for what it is via the tale of the Emperor's New Clothes, which represents the collective denial and double standards that are often a feature of social life. The apath in this context is someone who is willing to be blind, i.e. not to see that the Emperor is naked.

Apaths are an integral part of the sociopath's arsenal and contribute to sociopathic abuse; sociopaths have an uncanny knack of knowing who will assist them in bringing down the person they are targeting. It's not necessarily easy to identify an apath from the outside. In other circumstances an apath may show ample empathy and concern for others, just not in this case. The one attribute an apath must have is some connection to the sociopath's target.

Hence close friends, siblings, parents and other close relations can become accomplices to the sociopath and be instrumental in the downfall of the targeted individual.

How apaths, who may otherwise be fair-minded people, become involved in such destructive business isn't difficult to understand, though it can be hard to accept. The main qualifying attribute of the apath that renders him a willing accomplice is poor judgement resulting from lack of insight. This may be linked to reduced empathy for the targeted person. The apathetic person might bear a grudge, be jealous or angry, or have a sense of being let down by the individual concerned, and in consequence may be as keen as the sociopath to see the target defeated. Hence, the apath may be willing to join forces with the sociopath because he too has something to gain from the evolving situation.

At other times the apath doesn't want to see 'bad' in others, so chooses not to see it. On still other occasions, he might choose not to see because he has enough on his plate and doesn't possess the wherewithal or the moral courage to help the targeted person at that time. Usually, and whatever the reasons for his active or passive involvement, what happens during the course of interaction with a sociopath is that the apathetic person's conscience appears to fall asleep. Apaths walk in and out of situations in a trance-like state. It is this scenario that causes people blindly to follow leaders motivated only by self-interest. We excuse bullying, outrages, even murder, on the grounds that the leader knows best, regarding the injured and maimed targets not as fellow humans, but as objects, as 'it'.

This behaviour was demonstrated effectively in experiments carried out in the 1960s. In 1961–2, Yale University professor Stanley Milgram set up an experiment to test the human propensity to obey orders. A person playing the role of 'teacher' was given a list of word pairs which he was to teach the 'learner'. The teacher was then given an electric shock from an electro-shock generator as a sample of the shock that the learner would supposedly receive during the experiment. The teacher began the experiment by reading the list to the learner. The teacher then read the first word of each pair and read four possible answers.

The learner was asked to press a button to indicate his response. If the answer was incorrect, the teacher would administer a shock to the learner, with the voltage increasing in increments for each wrong answer. If correct, the teacher would read the next word pair. The subjects believed that for each wrong answer, the learner was receiving actual shocks. In fact there were no shocks.

During the experiment, many people indicated their desire to stop and check on the learner, and some paused to question the purpose of the experiment. But most continued after being assured that they wouldn't be held responsible. A few subjects began to laugh nervously or exhibit other signs of extreme stress after hearing 'staged' screams of pain coming from the learner. If the subject indicated he wanted to halt the experiment, he was given verbal instructions by the experimenter, in this order:

'Please continue.'
'The experiment requires that you continue.'
'It is absolutely essential that you continue.'
'You have no other choice, you must go on.'

If the subject still wished to stop after hearing all four instructions, the experiment was halted. Otherwise, it was stopped after the subject had been given the maximum 450-volt shock three times in succession. In the experiments, 62.5 per cent of the 'teachers' administered the experiment's final massive 450-volt shock, though many were very uncomfortable doing so.

Afterwards, Milgram summarized the experiment in an article titled 'The Perils of Obedience', declaring:

Ordinary people, simply doing their jobs, and without any particular hostility on their part, can become agents in a terrible destructive process. Moreover, even when the destructive effects of their work become patently clear and they are asked to carry out actions incompatible with fundamental standards of morality, relatively few people have the resources needed to resist authority.[1]

Milgram's experiments have been repeated many times over and yielded consistent results. What this evidence suggests is that a person of authority can strongly influence other people's behaviour. This is relatively useful in one way, as it makes it easy for an authority such as a government to establish order and control. But in the wrong hands such power and influence can have catastrophic consequences. The dubious nature of Milgram's experiments has attracted a great deal of ethical criticism, most importantly that he deceived the participants and didn't take adequate measures to protect them – indeed, within the context of this book, you might be forgiven for thinking such rather callous experiments have sociopathic tendencies. (Milgram's defence was that the results were unexpected and that their shocking nature, as much as the methods he used, may have evoked the criticisms.)

Apaths are portrayed in the 2008 film *The Wave* by German writer, actor and film director Dennis Gansel, in which high-school teacher Rainer Wenger sets out to examine the issue of autocracy in class. His students, the third generation after the Second World War, don't believe that a dictatorship could be established in modern Germany, so Wenger starts an experiment to demonstrate how easily the masses can be manipulated, rearranging the class on fascistic principles that include adopting a uniform, devising a salute and excluding nonconformists. Most of the students follow the new rules (i.e. they are apaths – people who blindly adhere to authority).

One student, however, Mona, leaves the group in disgust (in our view of things she is an **empath**, a category we will discuss next). The other classmates do not see any connection between their activity and fascism and believe that only good things have come from the movement. In fact, one young man, Tim (from our perspective an apath), becomes strongly committed to the group, offering to become Wenger's bodyguard. Wenger whips up the students' fervour as they continue to go along wholeheartedly with the new situation, but finally insists the Wave experiment must end and sends everyone home. But Tim produces a pistol and demands that everyone stays. He is desperate for the Wave to keep going because it has become his life. One of the other boys approaches him and Tim shoots him before turning the gun on himself.

This film, based on the book of the same name, was inspired in turn by the real-life social experiment the Third Wave, one of a number of 1960s studies that examined the disabling of conscience and human nature's tendency to adhere blindly to authority. The experiment was conducted in 1967 by teacher Ron Jones at Cubberley High School in Palo Alto, California. It was designed to demonstrate that democratic societies are not immune to the appeal of fascism.

What the aforementioned experiment and film indicate is that some people are more malleable than others. Importantly, they tell us that a greater number of us lack a backbone than perhaps we would like to think. In fact the studies suggest that over 60 per cent of us have a tendency to 'follow the leader', whether that leader is malign or benign. Within this majority group lurk the apaths, the foot-soldiers to the sociopath. Apaths are less able to see the situation for what it really is; their view of the bigger picture is obscured by their attitude to and opinion of the target, and by the sociopath's mesmeric influence.

Apaths are often fearful people; individuals who feel they do not possess the level of skill required to confront a challenge. They are the ones most likely to go with the flow, to agree that the Emperor is wearing new clothes. But apaths may also fail to perceive any threat at all. A danger is of no importance if one denies its existence. An apath's response to a sociopath's call to arms can then result from a state of 'learned helplessness'. Apaths behave defencelessly because they want to avoid unpleasant or harmful circumstances. Apathy is an avoidance strategy.

To shed more light on the behaviour of apaths we'll now relate some real-life stories. The first account comes from Nancy Ellen Iandoli, who survived life with a sociopathic mother and was left to face difficult times because of her father's inaction:

> My father was one of seven brothers. My mother was one of 14 children. Not one relative ever went out of their way to try and help me or even have me play with my cousins. Growing up I was very isolated as we didn't participate in holiday gatherings with any relatives. My mother always had a sour attitude and had complaints about everyone. No one visited us and I was trapped in my childhood hell with a sociopath mother and a loving father who worked all the time (partly to not have to be with his wife). I felt like an outcast from a very young age.
>
> My father was a World War Two veteran and spent four years in France, Germany and Austria. His troop liberated Dachau concentration camp. Post-traumatic stress disorder or PTSD was unknown in those days but I would say my father had PTSD, as he saw many atrocities. I think the combination of his childhood, with a stern and possibly abusive Italian immigrant father, and the war, meant that what emotions he experienced were held deep inside. I only saw my father cry twice in my life, when a good friend died and when he himself was dying. Whenever I sought his help about my sociopath mother, he would tell me to ignore her and not pay her attention as she was nuts like the rest of her family.

As a teenager, when I had a car, he would give me money for petrol and say go out with your friends and get away from her. He never divorced her as he didn't want to split his assets with her. But by not divorcing, he left me with a mess because eventually, after he died, my father's estate, the money he intended me to inherit, was stolen from me by a maternal cousin. I would say he felt helpless about the situation. I know they didn't divorce when I was younger because he didn't want my mother to use me as a pawn and he felt that leaving me with her 100 per cent of the time would be detrimental to my well-being.

I know he did the best he could, and I am not mad with my father at all. I don't know how he put up with my mother. I suppose he compensated for the situation at home by working a lot and by supporting his family financially, which was his socially accepted role. Dad and his six brothers ran a large corporation. Five of my uncles' families are taken care of financially but two of us have been done out of at least one million dollars. My father bought a house for me to live in with my little boy after I divorced and he bought a house for himself too because he couldn't tolerate his sociopathic wife. He was a solitary man who sought peace and quiet in his retirement years away from his wife.

When his estate was stolen by my maternal cousin, I sought out a couple of my maternal aunts and uncles and they did nothing. I sought out a couple of paternal cousins, but they did nothing. One cousin said he would pray for me! They didn't have their inheritance stolen. The toll of the abuse – both emotional and financial – has been harsh.

Another survivor of childhood sociopathic abuse is Colleen Fourie. Colleen experienced physical and emotional abuse at the hands of her mother. What compounded her unhappiness at home still further was her father's apparent inability to deal with the abuse. Here she discusses her father's apathy and possible reasons for it:

My father was one of seven, the eldest son. He grew up poor, as did many Afrikaners, having lost all their land in the Boer War. He only got an education by winning bursaries. He went to fight in the Second World War against his parents' wishes (his own father had been in a British concentration camp as a very small child and had lost a brother and a sister there) and he never really recovered from the experience. He was a pilot during the war, and suffered depression all his life from things he saw. He had a breakdown in London and spent a month or two in the Atkinson Morley Hospital, which is when my mother started taking lovers. Later he worked in the diplomatic corps.

I always worshipped my father. To me, he was 'The Good One'. He didn't spend much time with me, but what time he did was treasured for ever. In London, he made me a beautiful doll's house with real windows and a staircase. I watched closely and later made one for my own children, albeit out of cardboard! In Hamburg, he took me sailing, and we would go on long walks and drives, just exploring the country-side doing things like searching for the source of the Alster River.

When my mother was nasty to me, he would take me aside and explain that she hadn't been loved as a child, and that she didn't mean to hurt me, and really loved me, and that we must be very kind and understanding towards her. I only realized much later how harmful that was; it really set me up for my narcissist husband! Even as recently as a year ago, it dawned on me that although he took me sailing, I wore no life jacket. And I was allowed to sit right out on the prow. He took risks with my safety. One New Year's Eve, as we stood out in the snow on the large veranda of our flat, he put a firecracker in my hand. I remember my mother protesting, but he said it was safe – it said so on the packet. He lit it, and a few seconds later, it exploded in my hand. I nearly lost two fingers. I was rushed off to the Harbour Hospital where they special-ized in burns, and spent a couple of weeks there being spoilt rotten by the staff. So although I loved him, I couldn't really trust his judgement.

Later he developed a drinking problem. And then life became really complicated. My father let me down badly in the end – all those years he would tell me how I'd never have to worry about my children because he'd created an education fund for them. There was no such thing.

Turning a blind eye is a common trait of the apath, as this next account makes evident:

George

George, an apath, was so used to his sociopathic wife telling him what to do and what to say that he didn't see anything wrong in it. He learned to act defencelessly as a means of getting through life. Thus it became more or less a habit to turn a blind eye if his wife challenged or threatened others, even if the person targeted happened to be one of his children. The sociopathic wife bossed him about in order to keep control of her domain and possessions (these included family members, whom it has to be said she viewed as objects, not human beings). If she felt someone was getting too close to her foot-soldier husband, she would view them as a threat and start an offensive.

Her usual approach was to slyly make snide remarks and hurtful comments, or tell lies about a target's character. If the victim responded angrily, as naturally most would, she would turn to her husband and say 'See, George, I told you, she hates me', to which the husband would go along and lend support to her outrage. It is likely that the apath husband occasionally overheard the criticisms and accusations she directed at the targeted person but chose to ignore them. And she, accustomed to his passivity, had long ceased bothering to keep her remarks out of earshot. In the end he became so practised in self-trickery and so fearful of a showdown that he submissively went along with her every time.

In the case histories presented in Chapter 2, we see similar behaviour exhibited by Mary's loving but dispirited father in the story of the sociopathic parent, and we see Susan, the downtrodden wife of Peter our sociopathic spouse, adopt the apath role during the worst years of her marriage.

The empath

Not always, but quite often, the person targeted by the sociopath is an empath. To understand why this is, and what is going on when it happens, we first need to understand what an empath is. Most human beings have the ability to empathize, but some have more ability than others. Empathy is a vague and elusive concept. For US neuroscientist Jean Decety, empathy resembles 'a sort of minor constellation . . . stars glowing in the cosmos of an otherwise dark brain'. He is referring to the network of regions of the brain; the anterior cingulate cortex and anterior insula that light up orange on an fMRI scan when a person witnesses another in pain.[2] Yet empathy is more than orange-lit bits of brain. It is something that makes us human, or rather, humane.

Empathy is a shared emotion. To show empathy is emotionally to put yourself in the place of another. It is a learned phenomenon that requires emotional control and the capacity to distinguish oneself from others. Most of us possess the automatic ability to perceive and share others' feelings. A baby listening to another baby cry will cry too. Unconsciously people mimic the facial expressions of those they see. The ability to empathize is directly dependent on your ability to feel your own feelings and identify what they are. If you have never felt a certain feeling, it will be hard for you to understand how someone else is experiencing that feeling.

An empath, in the context that we apply the term, is not a person with near magical powers. Empaths are ordinary people who are highly perceptive and insightful and belong to the 40 per cent of human beings who sense when something's not right (those who respond to their 'gut instinct'). Going back to our folktale, 'The Emperor's New Clothes', the empath is the boy who mentions the unmentionable: that the Emperor isn't wearing any clothes.

Back in the 1990s, researchers suggested that there was a positive relationship between empathy and **emotional intelligence**.[3] Since then that term has been used interchangeably with **emotional literacy**. What this means in practice is that empaths have the ability to understand their own emotions, to listen to other people and empathize with their emotions, to express emotions productively and to handle their emotions in such a way as to improve their personal power.[4]

Empathy is a powerful communication tool that is often underused and undervalued in today's world. Yet the world needs as many empaths as it can find, for empaths are often mediators, go-betweens and peacemakers. Disharmony creates an uncomfortable feeling in an empath and in a confrontation he will try to settle things quickly. People are often attracted to empaths because of their compassionate nature. Even complete strangers find it easy to talk to empaths about personal matters because in general they make great listeners. A particular attribute of empaths is that they are sensitive to the emotional distress of others. Conversely they have trouble comprehending a closed mind and lack of compassion in others. They can be highly expressive and inclined to talk openly about themselves, although they often find it difficult to handle a compliment. Very highly empathetic people (sometimes termed super-empaths) may find themselves helping others at the expense of their own needs, which can lead them to withdraw from the outside world and become loners.

It's odd; most of us enjoy watching films and reading books about heroes who refuse to go along with the crowd, which suggests there is something admirable about people who make a bold stand, but in real life watching someone raise their head above the parapet often makes the rest of us feel queasy. Most – the 60 per cent plus majority – prefer the easy life and choose to maintain the status quo. What prevents many of us from acting on our consciences is fear; fear hems us in. It was interesting to discover, when doing the research for this book, how often people referred to empathetic types as fearful, too sensitive and vulnerable. In other words, many see empaths in problematical terms. It is true that some psychologists consider super-empathy a personality disorder or difficulty in its own right, especially if an individual reaches a state where he is so moved by others' emotions that he is overwhelmed by the amount of empathy he feels. But our experience suggests that people of such extreme empathy are few and far between. At any rate most empaths thrive very well in spite of, or indeed because of, their easy ability to empathize.

Empaths use their ability to empathize to boost theirs and others' well-being and safety. Problems arise for empaths, however, whenever there are apaths in the vicinity. Empaths can be brought down, distressed and forced into the position of the lone fighter by the inaction of more apathetic types around them. Here is a typical scenario involving an empath fighting unaided among apaths.

Cameron
Cameron spied a boy being bullied by a gang behind the cricket pavilion. Other boys must have witnessed the incident, as he saw several of them walk close by. Without hesitation Cameron shouted to the gang to stop kicking the boy. Cameron's friends, who had been laughing and poking fun at each other moments before, watched aghast and then one by one began to creep away from the scene. Suddenly the field was deserted and Cameron faced the gang alone. He couldn't walk away and leave the boy to get a kicking; his conscience would not allow it. So he braved their insults and name-calling and stood there, determined not to back down. The gang leader sensed his authority was weakened by Cameron's presence, so he told his bully-boys to let go of the victim: 'We'll get him later,' he said, 'when this ****'s not around to spoil things.' To Cameron's surprise and disappointment, when the boy was released from the gang's clutches, he was less than grateful that he had missed out on a beating. Cameron didn't know what infuriated him more: the boy's lack of gratitude or that his mates were nowhere to be seen.

The sociopathic transaction

Often empaths are targeted by sociopaths because they pose the greatest threat. The empath is usually the first to detect that something is not right and express what he or she senses. As a consequence, the empath is both the sociopath's number one foe and a source of attraction; the empath's responses and actions provide excellent entertainment for a bored and listless sociopath going about her daily business. Cameron's story highlights what happens to empaths who become embroiled in the intimidations of a bully.

The world of the empath is not for the fainthearted, and it is easy to see why others walk away from these kinds of confrontational situations. In the context that we are discussing, empaths often find themselves up against not only the sociopath but quite often a flock of apaths as well. Apaths hide among the 60 per cent of people who obediently follow the leader. On the basis of these traits they are afforded pole position in the sociopath's intrigues. But this prime spot comes at a price, for in what we call the **sociopathic transaction**, the apath makes an unspoken Faustian pact with the sociopath, and then passively (often through fear) or otherwise, participates in his cruel sport.

The Sociopath-Empath-Apath Triad

For a sociopathic transaction to be effective it requires the following threesome: a sociopath, an empath and an apath. We call this the **Sociopath-Empath-Apath Triad** – SEAT for short. The usual set-up goes something like this: the empath is forced to make a stand on seeing the sociopath say or do something underhand. The empath challenges the sociopath, who straight away throws others off the scent and shifts the blame on to the empath. The empath becomes an object of abuse when the apath corroborates the sociopath's perspective. Ultimately the situation usually ends badly for the empath, and sometimes also for the apath (if his conscience comes back to haunt him or subsequently he becomes an object of abuse himself). Frustratingly, however, the sociopath often gets off scot free.

Sociopaths rarely vary this tried and tested formula because it virtually guarantees them success. In fact, in almost every sociopathic interaction we know of, this interpersonal exchange is enacted. The sociopathic transaction relies heavily on the apathy of those close to the event or situation and highlights the importance of the apath in the transaction, as indicated in Figure 1 overleaf.

Sociopaths draw in apaths by numerous means: flattery, bribery, disorienting them with lies. A sociopath will go to any lengths to win her game. The best way to illustrate the interplay, and the ease with which apaths are pulled in, is by another short story.

Steve and Robin

Steve and Robin, both microbiologists at a prestigious university, were collaborators on an important vaccine trial. The head of department,

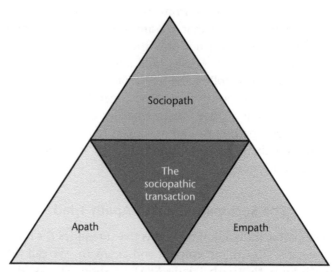

Figure 1   The Sociopath-Empath-Apath Triad (SEAT)

Ben, was the principal investigator. An arrogant and surly man in his early forties, he was a taskmaster and bully, though lauded by the university bigwigs because his reputation for excellent research helped secure large grants. With this new project he hoped to gain substantially; an important new vaccine could see his status in his field rise still further and prove the catalyst for a glittering scientific career.

His colleagues worked relentlessly on the trial collecting data. With the early phase over, Ben set about drafting a paper on their preliminary findings for submission to a respected scientific journal. Unbeknown to his colleagues, Ben decided that the outcome didn't look nearly as tantalizing as he had hoped, so he falsified some key results in order to present their findings in the best possible light. On completing the first draft he sent out the paper for comment to his colleagues. Steve replied immediately by email and confirmed he was happy with the manuscript. In fact he used the opportunity to suck up to his boss, thanking him for writing the paper so swiftly. Robin, on the other hand, was aghast. He read it over and over, noting what he saw as colossal errors. With great urgency, he rattled off an email to Ben.

Receiving no immediate response, he phoned Ben. When Ben didn't pick up, Robin went to find him in person, discovering him in the cafeteria with Steve. He was already too late, however. Ben had just been poisoning Steve's mind, saying that Robin had challenged him over the accuracy of the results due to a long-standing grudge rooted in his own inefficiency. Ben had, he said, had to pull Robin up about his own work several months back.

Steve, however, was different, Ben implied – much more thorough. He intimated that Steve would be on course for promotion: 'Especially if we get this paper out and secure funding for the next stage trials off of it.' By the time Robin joined them, Steve, though initially shocked, had already been won over by Ben's swift flattery and insinuations.

Seeing Ben and Steve together at a table, Robin crossed the cafeteria to them. 'Hi, you two got a moment?' Briefly there was an awkward silence. Steve exchanged a look with Ben, who gave a slight conspiratorial smile, now that the transaction was done and the sport under way. 'Yes, we've got a few moments. We were just talking about the paper. By the way I did see your email, but if you look at the paper thoroughly I think you'll find that everything is correct.' Robin turned to Steve to see how he was reacting to this nonsensical account of the situation. Steve looked at him with a smug look on his face. 'I'm with Ben on this one, Robin. There are no flaws in the analysis or the write-up of the study that I can see. We should be grateful Ben got it turned round so quickly.'

Robin was totally floored. 'You can't be serious? You're happy for it to go off to be reviewed with all these serious errors in it? Our reputations will be left in ruins when this gets out.'

Robin decided to make a stand. He asked for his name to be removed as a co-author of the paper but was exasperated to learn that it was sent off to the journal anyway. More frustratingly still, it was published within a few months. Meanwhile the workplace became a source of stress for Robin as he struggled to cope with the backlash from colleagues who saw his intervention as an attempt to sabotage their work. People avoided him at break times, and when they did talk to him, the conversation was awkward and stilted.

Eventually Robin arranged a meeting with Ben to have it out once and for all. But when the time came for the meeting Ben took control of the agenda. 'Robin, I have to be honest with you, many of your colleagues are unhappy about the way you handled things and some have made complaints about the standard of your recent work. Furthermore your colleagues don't trust you to conduct yourself professionally after you attempted to sabotage their hard work. Mercifully the reviewers saw what a damn fine trial we'd conducted and didn't get wind of your attempted slur. We can't afford to have a saboteur on the team, someone so reckless they would put the whole research project at risk. So I've discussed this with the Dean and he agrees there's no future for you here, and no other way to deal with this. You've got to go.'

The 'gaslighting' effect and how it works

Let's now explain the sociopath's standard mode of operation. According to Martha Stout, sociopaths frequently use **gaslighting** tactics. In our story Ben (the sociopath) targets Robin (the empath) and uses Steve (the apath) as a corroborator in the abuse. The actions of both Ben and Steve have a 'gaslighting' effect on Robin.

Gaslighting is the systematic attempt by one person to erode another's reality. The syndrome gets its name from the 1938 stage play *Gas Light* (originally known as *Angel Street* in the USA), and the 1940 and 1944 film adaptations. The 1944 film *Gaslight* features a murderer who attempts to make his wife doubt her sanity. He uses a variety of tricks to convince her that she is crazy, so she won't be believed when she reports the strange things that are genuinely occurring, including the dimming of the gas lamps in the house (which happens when her husband turns on the normally unused gas lamps in the attic to conduct clandestine activities there). The term has since found its way into clinical and research literature.

Gaslighting is a form of psychological abuse in which false information is presented in such a way as to make the target doubt his or her own memory and perception. Psychologists call this, rather incongruously, 'the sociopath's dance'. It may simply involve the denial by an abuser that previous abusive incidents ever occurred, or it could be the staging of strange events intended to disorientate the target. In any event, the effect of gaslighting is to arouse such an extreme sense of anxiety and confusion in the target that he reaches the point where he no longer trusts his own judgement. The techniques are similar to those used in brainwashing, interrogation and torture, the instruments of psychological warfare. This is Machiavellian behaviour of the worst kind. A target exposed to it for long enough loses her sense of her own self. She finds herself second-guessing her own memory, becomes depressed and withdrawn and totally dependent on the abuser for her sense of reality.

Gaslighting is a deliberate ploy that occurs between one individual (the **gaslighter** – the sociopath in our case) and another (the **gaslightee**, often an empath). The endgame for the sociopath is when the gaslightee thinks he is going crazy. Anyone can become the victim of a sociopath's gaslighting moves. Gaslighting can take place in any kind of relationship – between parent and child, between siblings or friends, or between groups of people including work colleagues. Going back to our analogy of the Emperor's New Clothes, it is the process of gaslighting that distorts our sense of reality and makes us disbelieve what we see. Even when the victim is bewildered there is a reluctance to see the gaslighter for what he is. Denial is essential for gaslighting to work.

Psychotherapist Christine Louis de Canonville describes different phases that the abuser leads the relationship through: the **idealization** stage, the **devaluation** stage and the **discarding** stage.[5] Gaslighting does not happen all at once, so if you suspect in the early stages of a relationship that you are being gaslighted, you can protect yourself by walking away. However, you need to be informed as to what those stages look like to make that choice. Let's now explore them briefly.

The idealization stage

During this early stage the sociopath shows herself in the best possible light. But this phase is an illusion. The sociopath intends only to draw her target in. At the beginning of the relationship she is usually ultra-attentive, charming, energetic, exciting and great fun. If the context is a new romantic relationship, the targeted person may feel he loves the sociopath intensely. It can feel like an addictive or hypnotic sort of love. Caught up in the euphoria, he becomes hooked. If the context is a friendship, the person targeted may feel she has never in her life met anyone with whom she has more in common. In the workplace, the person may feel she has finally found a boss who sees her true potential. The target does all he or she can to gain the sociopath's special approval. The boss might tempt him along with words to the effect of 'I see a lot of me in you'.

The devaluation stage

Once the sociopath has assessed the target's strengths and weaknesses, the first phase is over and the devaluation stage begins. From here on in, the sociopath is cold and unfeeling. This phase begins gradually so the targeted person is not alert to the transformation. Nevertheless at some point it will begin to seem to the target that he can't do anything right. She feels devalued at every turn. Totally confused, the targeted person becomes increasingly stressed, unhappy, low in mood or depressed. The gaslighting effect is under way. Confused by the sociopath's behaviour, the targeted person tries harder to please his sociopathic abuser in order to get the relationship back on track. But no matter what he does, he only seems to cause the sociopath further injury. The target gets caught up in a spiral of socio-pathic abuse where unpredictability and uncertainty are routine, until finally he becomes a shadow of his former self. The paradox of the situation is that the more distressed the target becomes, the more the sociopath enjoys the power of the situation, and the more powerful she feels, the more blatant and extreme her abuse becomes.

Devaluation, according to Louis de Canonville, can be delivered through many different forms and levels of attack. The targeted person has been conditioned, appearing in all intents and purposes to the outside world to be a willing partner in the sociopath's games. If he does manage to escape the sociopathic individual, he is at high risk of future entrapment by other sociopaths, because he is primed in a way that other sociopaths can spot.

The discarding stage

In the discarding stage, the game comes to its conclusion. By this time the sociopath has lost her ardour for the game, for she views the contest as already won. The target is reduced to an object, something to which the sociopath is totally indifferent; it is as if the targeted individual no longer exists. The targeted person on the other hand is left confused and raw with emotion. In the context of a romantic association he may scrabble around trying to find a way to rescue the dying relationship. But the sociopath resists all attempts to re-establish any connection, using bullying tactics such as silence or coldness in retaliation; she is probably already making moves to secure her next target.

The effects of gaslighting from the targeted person's point of view

During the process of gaslighting, the targeted person usually goes through some recognizable emotional and psychological states of mind. Psychologist Dr Robin Stern describes three stages those tar-geted go through: disbelief, defence and depression.[6]

Disbelief

The targeted person's initial reaction to gaslighting behaviour is one of complete disbelief; he cannot believe the sudden change towards him, or that he is being gaslighted. All he knows is that something terribly distressing seems to be happening, but he can't figure out what. Blinded by the sociopath's promises or affections, the targeted person naturally trusts that his friendship or love is returned, but of course, this belief is based upon falsehood. In consequence the sociopath offers no sympathy or support when the target seeks to put the relationship right. Gaslighting doesn't need to be severe in order to have stark effects on the gaslighted person. It can be as subtle as being told 'You are so sensitive' or having it suggested that you are incapable: for example, 'You can't do that. You'll have to leave it to me.' Even though the targeted person knows on a rational level that these statements are untrue, his confidence is so eroded that he can't trust his own view. In extreme cases, those desperate for reassurance that they're not going mad become very dependent on their abuser for a sense of reality.

Defence

In the early stages of the devaluation phase the targeted person still has the emotional wherewithal to defend himself against the manipulation. However, at some point he is thrown off balance by creeping self-doubt, anxiety and guilt. Becoming bewildered and unable to trust his own instincts or memory, he tends to isolate himself because of the shame he feels. Eventually he is left unable to defend himself from the unbearable gaslighting effect.

One psychological condition that can result is called **Stockholm syndrome**. This got its name from a 1973 bank robbery in Stockholm, Sweden, when four bank employees were strapped in dynamite and locked in a vault. Much to their rescuers' surprises, the hostages developed more trust in their captors than in the police who were trying to rescue them. The term was subsequently coined by Swedish psychiatrist and criminologist Nils Bejerot, who was involved in the case. Stockholm syndrome can occur in situations where people find themselves held captive and in fear of their lives – not only thanks to sociopathic abuse but in kidnapping and hostage situations. It refers to the way in which someone in such a situation may bond with his or her captor as a defence mechanism – what

is technically known as **traumatic bonding**. In order to cope with
the discomfort of living in such madness and chaos, the targeted
person – and apaths too if they are involved long enough – cope
by rationalizing and excusing the sociopath's behaviour in order to
reduce the conflict they are experiencing. Louis de Canonville calls
it a 'clever, but complicated unconscious' self-preservation strategy.

Depression

By the time someone has been systematically gaslighted, he hardly
recognizes himself. In fact many such people become a shadow of
their former selves. They begin to feel that they can't do anything
right any more, that they don't feel that they can trust their own
mind or trust the opinion of others. So they withdraw into a distorted version of what is really taking place. Some escape into a
state of constant low mood or depression. Depression is different
from normal sadness – it is worse, as it affects the person's physical
health and it goes on for longer. A lot of people who have been
gaslit for a sustained period in this way go on to experience post-
traumatic stress disorder (see Chapter 5 for more on this). This is
especially true of children of sociopathic parents.

In the aftermath of sociopathic abuse people may experience an
array of responses – shock, disbelief, deep sadness, guilt, shame,
anger, fear, loneliness and an array of physical symptoms including
panic attacks, flashbacks, anxious thoughts, fatigue and dissociation – although many also express relief at finally knowing what has
been going on. Confidence erosion is another symptom that follows
constant gaslighting. Gaslighted individuals live in fear of doing the
wrong thing and making their situation even more dangerous. They
become more cautious and doubt themselves. This often affects
how they make decisions in their life. They commonly ask 'Am I too
sensitive?', 'Why do I attract people like this?' or 'Am I to blame?'

Shame and blame are the hallmarks of gaslighting. The targeted
person may become hyper-sensitive after the constant humiliation.
He hears countless times from the sociopath and her foot-soldier
apaths that he is 'too sensitive', so over time he begins to believe
these lies about himself.

Another negative side effect of having been gaslighted is that the
targeted person finds herself always apologizing, even for her very
existence. This is, to all intents and purposes, a way of avoiding

more conflict with the sociopath. Many children of sociopathic parents have a tendency to do this. It is not an act of politeness. Rather, as Christine Louis de Canonville argues, it is a powerful strategy for staying safe, and a means of disarming the sociopath.

One more knock-on effect that must be faced as a result of having experienced gaslighting is the resulting joylessness, a melancholic view of life. Many people who have experienced the traumatic effects of gaslighting go through such physical and mental tortures that they suffer a personality change. They may end up feeling confused, lonely, frightened and unhappy. But rather than expose their vulnerability they hold on to it and keep their feelings in. Targeted individuals often experience great shame about their situation. When well-meaning friends and family members show concern or ask whether they are OK, they avoid the subject and withhold information in order to avoid further pain.

Shame in sociopathic abuse is a difficult issue. The shame that a targeted person feels is a normal response to the sense of failure she feels as a result of her inability to protect herself (and her dependents) from abuse. In addition, other people often have a 'blame the victim' mentality or take the attitude that the targeted person should 'just get over it', both of which demoralize the individual concerned. This shame can be interpreted by others as defensiveness, but in reality it is likely that the individual wishes to withdraw and socially isolate herself out of fear and lack of trust of others.

Some people who have been gaslighted also experience difficulty in making simple decisions. Having to ask permission to do anything, not being allowed to express their own opinion, never being able to win an argument, constantly being chastised and humiliated, contributes to a loss of their autonomy, even their ability to make decisions for themselves. Many individuals recovering from sociopathic abuse adopt 'people pleasing' behaviour as a way of coping and dealing with others. The reason is that, as a defence mechanism, the targeted person has become conditioned to please the sociopath. Sadly, the only person the targeted empath does not set out to please is himself. The behavioural and emotional difficulties that follow abuse at the hands of a sociopath mean that, for the unfortunate few who have endured years of such abuse, life can seem rather hopeless. In Chapter 5 we will discuss strategies for coping and turning things around.

5

Coping in the aftermath of a destructive relationship

When a sociopath performs his cruel play, take your cue and exit the stage.

(Fin McGregor)

That people can survive sociopathic abuse is testament to the fortitude of the human spirit. In this chapter we will discuss what it takes to stop sociopathic abuse in its tracks and get your life back.

Witnessing sociopathic abuse

So what should you do if you are aware that sociopathic abuse is taking place? If your brush with a sociopath is only fleeting, or you have witnessed someone else being abused, you will probably feel inclined to cease contact with the sociopath with immediate effect. But if you or someone else has been or remains in danger, you need to think about your obligation to report what you have experienced or witnessed to the police and other relevant agencies. In this way, you may prevent the same problem happening again. Evidence from victims and witnesses is important because it demonstrates the distress and damage that sociopathic behaviour can do in our communities. Apathy equates to collusion, so turning a blind eye is no option for a person of integrity.

Yet, in reality, many of us do find it hard to get involved. One of the barriers to speaking out is that sociopaths often work on evoking other people's pity. You should never agree to help a sociopath conceal his or her true identity, whether out of pity or for any other reason. If you find yourself pitying someone who consistently hurts you or other people, and who actively seeks your sympathy, the chances are you are dealing with a sociopath. The best advice is not to listen. In *The Sociopath Next Door*, Martha Stout stresses that while there is still interaction between you and the sociopath, it is best to resist the temptation to join in his games. Trying to outsmart the sociopath or getting into arguments with him reduces you to his level – and distracts you from the task of protecting yourself. It is better to resist a showdown with a sociopath at all costs. In such situations his drive to win sets in. The best way to protect yourself is to avoid him, and refuse any kind of contact or communication. Sociopaths feel no obligation to you or anyone else. To keep a sociopath in your life is therefore to put yourself at risk of harm.

If you find it difficult to exclude the sociopath from your life, it might help to remind yourself that by doing so you won't hurt anyone's feelings. Sociopaths' emotional repertoire is so limited that they don't have feelings to hurt. So look at the situation dispassionately. If you find that your family, friends and acquaintances have difficulty understanding why you want to avoid a particular individual, and put unwanted pressure on you to continue the relationship, don't give in. Remain unmoved by those who don't comprehend the danger of the situation, and have the strength of your convictions.

If total avoidance is out of the question, for instance if the sociopath is someone you work with, limit contact as much as possible. Above all, make the rules of engagement ones that are right for you and then do your utmost to stick to them. View the boundaries on contact as non-negotiable and turn a deaf ear to those who ask for explanations. Conversely, don't be afraid to be unsmiling or serious when explaining your position.

At some point most of us learn that we can't control other people's behaviour. This is important to keep at the forefront of your mind, as is the crucial point that the sociopath's behaviour is not your fault. It is far better to concentrate on your own behaviour and with sorting out your own life than to bother with things that you can't change.

Dealing with the draining effects of trauma

If you have been on the receiving end of direct and/or sustained sociopathic abuse, you may feel confused and bewildered in the aftermath. This section is intended to help you deal with the initial trauma and help you get back on your feet.

The very first steps towards recovery involve recognizing and accepting that abuses have occurred and taking steps to remove the sociopath from your life, or severely limit her influence. Recognizing and accepting the abuser and the abuse for what they are is a vital first step. Doing so helps draw the issue to the surface and lets you see and make sense of what has been happening to you.

If talking openly and directly to someone is too difficult at first, then 'talking to oneself' is a pretty good start. 'Talking to oneself' includes identifying useful self-help books, and searching the internet for online support groups and useful blogs (see the 'Useful addresses' section). Online groups can provide instant support and advice, as well as the chance to practise a new and stronger voice to be incorporated with your real-life identity over time. Online groups also provide a level of anonymity, though it is important to protect your privacy, especially if you are feeling especially vulnerable and at a crisis point in your life. So a word or two of caution about use of the internet: only discuss things you are willing to share and leave available in the public domain. Many online groups, such as those on Facebook, operate privacy policies and have operational policies in place to regulate proceedings, but sociopaths and other anti-social types love to lurk online, manifesting themselves as internet trolls (people who post inflammatory or insulting messages in an online community such as a forum, chat room or blog). Therefore the message to take on board is this: keep your wits about you, trust and respond to your gut instincts and proceed with caution.

Identifying the problem can seem a mammoth task at first. In the aftermath of sociopathic abuse individuals can feel such an extreme sense of anxiety and confusion that they no longer trust their own judgement. Entering a sociopathic relationship is a one-sided and isolating experience. On exiting a sociopathic relationship the isolation can be magnified as the abused person withdraws from social activities and becomes cut off from support. This is often the result of the immense shame abused people feel on account of their disempowerment, and their maltreatment by the sociopath in their lives.

Shame

In our experience, shame is the greatest barrier for individuals trying to move on. Shame and a growing wariness of others can make it hard for such people to open up about the true extent of their unhappy situation. The situation becomes more desperate if earlier attempts to gain understanding have been met with incredulity. Wariness coupled with deep and toxic shame can render the abused person inactive. Children, for instance, often learn from bitter experience that telling someone else about abuse at home can result in negative, even detrimental reactions.

Most of the time shame is a normal and healthy human emotion. A healthy sense of shame keeps our feet on the ground, and reminds us of the boundaries. We are human and we make mistakes. Feeling shame is giving ourselves permission to be human. A healthy amount of shame can deepen our sense of personal power, helping us to recognize our limits and learn to redirect our energies to more fruitful pursuits. But too much shame and for too long can be harmful and demoralizing. John Bradshaw, author of *Healing the Shame that Binds You*,[1] calls this toxic shame and argues that it can become a central part of oneself, leading to profound feelings of isolation. It is internalized emotion that can lead us to feel defective, beyond remedy.

It is not uncommon for people who experienced the shame and deprivation that goes with having a sociopath in the family to face difficulties in their adult relationships. Individuals who have experienced trauma at the hands of a sociopath in childhood may unwittingly seek out or attract needy and narcissistic types of people in adulthood. Shame in the children of sociopaths can be intense and hard to shake off, for it originates from the trauma of abandonment as a child.

In her powerful book, *The Drama of the Gifted Child*,[2] Alice Miller describes the notion of **abandonment trauma**. This type of trauma occurs when damage is caused as a result of something not happening to an individual (for example not feeling loved, nurtured or protected). We can't do justice to Miller's body of work in such a short book as this, but we do recommend those interested to read her work (see 'Further reading and resources'). In essence, being abandoned by a sociopathic parent who is physically present but emotionally absent can leave a child bewildered to the point of despair. In order to develop as healthy human beings, children need to mirror the actions of an adult carer who is both physically and emotionally present. A baby is completely dependent on its parents and the parents' love and care is essential. Denied his or her basic needs, a child must find ways not to be abandoned. Many children in this situation try to reverse the natural order: they take care of their parents, as opposed to the other way round. But this often leads to a paradoxical situation where the child is nevertheless abandoned.

Many children of sociopathic, neglectful parents try to make recompense by becoming caregivers. This can lead to excessive concern with pleasing and paying disproportionate attention to the care of others, at the expense of a proper concentration on oneself. Overwhelmingly, the children or partners of sociopaths tend to put others' needs first. They may feel they deserve the pain and trauma that goes with living with a sociopath; they usually rationalize that, after all, it was they and no one else that got them into this mess. This sort of thinking has a circularity about it, and if not interrupted and eventually terminated may drive a person near crazy.

Coping emotionally

The decision to change a situation of sociopathic abuse can be slow and laborious, or it may be experienced in a 'Eureka!' moment. One barrier to seeing the situation for what it is – abuse and trauma – is lack of self-confidence and self-belief, or fear of 'going it alone'; another might be that the relationship is a long-term one with children involved. In that case the timing and nature of the departure from the relationship can matter greatly. All the same, one day the abused person will find the courage to break free, or the sociopath in his or her life will walk out, probably without warning and leaving a whole lot of debris in his wake. Suddenly all alone, the abused person is left to contend with his or her grief and loss.

This phase can be bewildering and frightening. People react differently and take different lengths of time to come to terms with what has happened. Even so, you may be surprised by the strength of your feelings. It is normal to experience a mix of feelings. You may feel:

- *frightened* . . . that the same thing will happen again, or that you might lose control of your feelings and break down;
- *helpless* . . . that something really bad happened and you could do nothing about it. You feel vulnerable and overwhelmed;

- *angry* . . . about what has happened and with whoever was responsible;
- *guilty* . . . you may feel that you could have done something to prevent it;
- *sad* . . . particularly if you or other people (your children perhaps) have been affected;
- *ashamed or embarrassed* . . . that you have these strong feelings you can't control, especially if you need others to support you;
- *relieved* . . . that the danger is over and that the cause of the danger has gone;
- *hopeful* . . . that your life will return to normal. People often start to feel more positive about things quite soon after a trauma.

We liken the process to that of grieving. How we cope depends on our unique temperament and circumstances, but predictable stages of grief tend to follow.

Stages of grieving

Following a trauma of any magnitude many of us experience various stages of grief. We don't necessarily go through the stages one by one, in a neat linear way, and there is no typical response to loss. Grief is as individual as our lives. The most commonly recognized stages, as defined by Elisabeth Kübler-Ross, are denial, anger, bargaining, depression and acceptance.[3] Not everyone goes through all of them, or in that order, but knowing about the common experiences and stages of grief can equip us to cope better when we do experience them.

Denial

According to Kübler-Ross and Kessler, the first stage of grieving is concerned with surviving the loss. In this stage, the world becomes meaningless and overwhelming. Life makes no sense. We are in a state of shock and denial. We go numb. We wonder how we can go on. We find it difficult simply to get through each day. These are survival tactics that help to pace our feelings of grief. It is 'nature's way' of letting in only as much as we can handle. As we accept the reality of the loss, we start to ask questions and, unknowingly, begin the healing process. Without being aware of it we become a little stronger day by day, and the denial begins to fade. It is only as we proceed that all the feelings come to the surface, by which time we should be better equipped to handle them.

Anger

Anger is a necessary stage of the healing process. Be willing and unafraid to feel your anger, even though it may seem endless. The more you truly feel it, the more it will begin to dissipate and the more you will heal. There are many other emotions beneath the anger, and you will get to them in time, but anger is the emotion we are most used to managing. The truth is that anger has no bounds. It can extend not only to the sociopath who has left your life but also to your friends and your family, and to yourself.

Beneath anger is often pain. It is natural to feel pain at being deserted and abandoned, but we live in a society that fears anger. You may get angry at others now that you are no longer with the sociopath. Your anger is a driving force, something that has the propensity to propel you forward, and in that sense it is your ally, your friend. A connection made from the strength of anger feels better than nothing, so sometimes it is something we hold on to. We usually know more about suppressing anger than feeling it. The anger is just another indication of the intensity of your grief and sense of loss.

Bargaining

After a loss, bargaining may take the form of a temporary respite. Kübler-Ross and Kessler suggest that our conversations become full of 'If only . . .' or 'What if . . .' statements, such as 'What if I wake up and realize this has all been a bad dream?' We want life to be returned to what it was; we want it restored. The 'if onlys' cause us to find fault in ourselves and what we think we could have done differently. We are often willing to do anything not to feel the pain of a loss. In this state we may drink too much alcohol, take prescribed medication or illicit drugs to dampen or dull our senses, and we may eat too much or find whatever other means we can to block the pain. But doing so means we remain in the past, trying to circumvent the hurt.

Depression

After bargaining, our attention switches from the past to the here and now. Empty feelings may present themselves, and we may experience grief on a deeper level. This stage feels as though it will last for ever. It is important to understand that this depression or period of low mood is not a sign of mental illness but an appropriate response to loss. We withdraw from life and feel intense sadness.

Depression after a loss is too often seen as unnatural: a state to be fixed, something to snap out of. The first question to ask yourself is whether or not the situation you are in is actually depressing and if so, whether depression is a normal and appropriate response. Not to experience some level of depression would be unusual after a marriage or family breakdown or an extreme emotional assault. Once you are fully able to take in the nature of the loss, the realization of what you have experienced is understandably depressing. Thus we may need to accept that if grief is a process of healing, then depression is one of the many necessary steps along the way.

Acceptance

Acceptance is often confused with the notion of being 'all right' or 'OK' about a given situation, or of finding a place where one is able to forgive the other person (in our case the sociopath and/or his apathetic followers) for what has happened. This is not what we mean when we use the term acceptance here. Most people never reach a point of feeling all right about the losses and traumas they have experienced. What this stage is about is accepting the reality of the situation and recognizing that this new reality is permanent; in other words arriving at a point where we learn to live with it and where living with it becomes the new norm. In resisting the new norm, people cling to the hope of maintaining life as it was before. In time, however, we come to see that we can't maintain the past in the present. It has been changed and we must adjust. Hence we learn to accept new roles for ourselves and others.

Finding acceptance may simply entail having more good days than bad ones. We can't replace our old lives and relationships, but we can make new connections and meaningful new relationships. Instead of denying our feelings, we must listen to our needs in order to move, change, grow and evolve. Once grief has been given its rightful stint, this is a time to live again.

Dealing with anxiety, stress and anger in the early days

Anxiety, stress and anger may result from continued association with a sociopath, or from the process of grieving for the relationship you thought you had with the sociopath before you discovered it was phoney. Left unchecked, anxiety and stress can build up and lead to anxiety disorders. When we become stressed or angry, our body's levels of fight-or-flight hormones such as cortisol and adrenalin increase. If we don't then either run or fight, the cortisol and adrenalin stay in the body, affecting the immune system, sleep and emotional well-being. These hormones have been linked with both heart disease and depression. We estimate that a sizeable amount of referrals to psychiatric services for anxiety disorders and depression arise from circumstances involving sociopathic abuse. To prevent this occurring to you, it is important to deal with anxiety and find ways to manage it.

If you find you have a particular problem with stress and anger, this section of the book may help you. Here we'll examine some techniques that may help you manage stress and anger in the early days after suffering a trauma.[4]

Pressing the pause button

The first step is to press the pause button and buy some time out from your anger and frustration. You might want to ask yourself the following questions:

- *What will I do to press the pause button?*
  You might try walking away, counting to ten, distracting yourself, keeping quiet or just biting your tongue.
- *What things might I try to stop me getting angry?*
  Possibilities include breathing, self-talk, exercise, talking to someone you trust, assertiveness.

One way to look at situations in which you easily get angry is by dividing up your thoughts into hot and cool ones. For example:

Hot thoughts	*Cool thoughts*
How dare he!	Don't let it wind you up
She's trying to humiliate me	I probably don't have all the facts
It's the same things over again	It might be different this time

It can be difficult to identify your thoughts, so another way of looking at the issue is to view thoughts as 'self-talk', or talking things over in your head. This is a normal thing to do and it can be really helpful. You can use self-talk to help when you are going into a difficult situation in which you may possibly get angry. You can also use it to get through a difficult situation, or to review what you did afterwards.

Tips for tackling stress

There are hundreds if not thousands of books on dealing with stress or anxiety, but to keep things simple here are our top ten tips for tackling stress, adapted from those of the UK mental health charity, MIND:[5]

1 *Make the connection.* Could the fact that you're feeling 'not right' be a response to what the sociopath has put you through?
2 *Take a regular break.* Give yourself a brief break whenever you feel things are getting on top of you.
3 *Learn to relax.* Follow a simple routine to relax your muscles and slow your breathing.
4 *Get better organized.* Make a list of the problems you need to tackle and deal with one task at a time.
5 *Sort out your worries.* Divide them into those that you can do something about (either now or soon) and those that you can't. There's no point in worrying about things that you can't change.
6 *Change what you can.* Look at the problems that can be resolved, and get whatever help is necessary to sort them out. Learn to say 'no'.
7 *Look at your long-term priorities.* What can you off-load, or change? How can you get your life into better balance?
8 *Improve your lifestyle.* Find time to eat properly, get plenty of exercise and enough sleep. Avoid drinking and smoking too much. However much you believe they can help you to relax, they tend to have the opposite effect.
9 *Confide in someone.* Don't keep your emotions bottled up.
10 *Focus on the positive aspects of your life.*

Relaxation exercise

And here is a set of simple instructions to help you learn to relax:

1 Close your eyes and breathe slowly and deeply.
2 Locate any areas of tension and try to relax the muscles involved; imagine the tension disappearing.
3 Relax each part of your body, in turn, from your feet to the top of your head.
4 As you focus on each part of your body, think of warmth, heaviness and relaxation.
5 After 20 minutes, take some deep breaths and stretch your body.

Frustration

People with anger difficulties often talk about first becoming frustrated, and getting angry after the frustration sets in. Frustration is an emotion that we all experience from time to time. It develops when you are thwarted or hindered while trying to do something or reach a goal. It is the feeling you get when you expect a different outcome from what really happens. Although frustration can be helpful, as it leads to new ways of thinking about a problem, it is basically about not getting what we want, or getting what we don't want. Finding ways to manage frustration may improve our sense of well-being in everyday life.

There are a variety of factors that can trigger frustration. These include:

- **thoughts** – unrealistic expectations, plans, ideas for yourself or others (such thoughts may include the words *should, must, ought*: 'she *should* do what I told her');
- **situations** – particular places or tasks you would rather avoid;
- **relationships** – contact with people you would prefer not to see.

Frustration tolerance

Frustration often occurs when we have expectations for ourselves or others that are too high, or that are simply unattainable. In such cases we may have to alter our perspective or way of thinking. We may need to become what is called in the world of therapeutics **frustration tolerant**. To be frustration tolerant is to continue living a balanced, healthy life despite encountering repeated interferences and obstacles. How frustration tolerant we are refers to how robust we are in the face of life's stressors and challenges. If someone gets easily frustrated when she cannot get what she wants, she is said to have low frustration tolerance. Her frustration is intolerable and she can't cope. This way of thinking leads to the discomfort being increased. People with low frustration tolerance underestimate their ability to cope with discomfort (they might say 'I can't bear it!' or 'I can't stand it!'). Describing something as 'intolerable' frequently makes situations appear more daunting or off-putting than they actually are.

We can stand frustrating times if we choose to think about these situations in a different way. Therefore the best approach might be to find ways of controlling the degree of frustration that we experience in daily life. This may be achieved by changing the things we do, or thoughts we have, when we feel frustrated. Alternatively, if there is nothing we can do, it may consume less energy if we are able to learn to accept and tolerate the uncomfortable experiences.

The most effective approach to overcoming low frustration is to develop an attitude of high frustration tolerance. This is the ability to tolerate discomfort while waiting to get what you want. Basically it is about toughing things out. Increasing tolerance for frustration helps us to experience normal levels of healthy annoyance in response to being blocked. High frustration tolerance enables people to be more effective at solving problems or accepting things that, at least at present, cannot be changed.

Examples of high frustration tolerance statements are:

- 'This is an uncomfortable situation but I can stand the discomfort.'
- 'This situation is hard to bear but I can bear it – some difficult things are worth tolerating.'
- 'Even if I feel like I can't take it any more, past experience has shown that I probably can.'

To increase your frustration tolerance, ask these types of questions:

- 'Can I remember being in this situation before and coping with it?'
- 'Is it true that I can't stand this situation or is it just that I don't like this situation?'
- 'Is this situation truly unbearable or is it really just very difficult to bear?'

Being less extreme in our judgement of negative situations can help us have less extreme emotional responses, such as energy-depleting anger. Many situations are difficult to tolerate, but we need to remember at such times that we have tolerated similar situations in the past.

Venting

'Venting' means releasing pent-up feelings of anger or getting things off your chest. Venting is often explosive and can be an act of aggression. When people vent their anger, they often feel better immediately afterwards. However, not long after that, most people report feeling guilty, ashamed or sad for the hurt that they caused another person. Originally venting was thought to be helpful and healthy for reducing anger difficulties. However, recent evidence suggests that venting is not healthy because it increases the chances of further anger in the future.

Reducing venting

The following steps may help you express your anger in a healthier way:

1 Recognize and label your angry feelings: 'I am feeling angry because . . .'
2 Is the incident that has made you angry important or unimportant?
3 If it is important, can you influence or control it?
4 If it is important and you can control it, are there strategies you can use to implement the actions? If so, then list them. If it is not important, dismiss it and move on.

Rumination

Rumination involves dwelling on or thinking deeply about something. Everybody does it from time to time, but some forms of rumination can be unhealthy for us to indulge. People ruminate by bringing thoughts, memories and imagined events to mind and going over and over them. This can have a negative impact on our mental health. Ruminating about the darker side of life can lead to anxiety, depression and anger. Rumination can impair thinking, motivation, concentration, memory and problem-solving, and can drive away people who might be willing to support us. It can also increase stress. There are several types of rumination:

- **Anxious rumination.** When people worry, they go over thoughts about bad things that might happen to them or others. People with social anxiety go over what others might think of them, and over things they think they've done wrong in a certain situation. People with health anxiety think that they have serious illnesses.
- **Depressive rumination** involves dwelling on the causes and consequences of feeling depressed (lack of motivation or hopelessness). Depression can be related to a fear of anger, and ruminating can arise from fear of hurting others.
- **Anger rumination** may focus on injustice, angry memories, thoughts of revenge or angry afterthoughts. The way we think about things affects our emotions and our bodies. If, for example, you are hungry and see your favourite meal, your mouth will water. Nonetheless, just thinking or imagining your favourite meal will have a similar effect, because our thoughts stimulate areas of the brain responsible for digestion. Likewise, ruminating about something will trigger the fight-or-flight response and get our bodies psyched up.

Know yourself

What happens when you ruminate or dwell on negative events? It helps to think about the physical, behavioural and emotional effects. What do you ruminate about? What are the usual triggers? What are the consequences? As with all aspects of anger, the first task is to recognize *when* you are doing it. So whenever you start to dwell on something that makes you feel angry, remind yourself that you are ruminating – 'WARNING! I'm ruminating' – and stop as quickly as possible. If ruminating has become a habit, however, this may be easier said than done. And as with all habits, patience and practice of new behaviours are essential.

1 When you find yourself dwelling on what has happened, say to yourself, 'Stop ruminating!'
2 Calm yourself by breathing, relaxation, meditation or exercise.
3 Question the purpose and value of ruminating. Ask yourself:
   - Would I advise a friend to think in this way?
   - What would a friend say to me if she knew I was ruminating?

- Am I looking at the whole picture?
- Does it really matter that much?
- What would I say about this in five years' time? Will it be that important?
- Do I apply one set of rules or standards to myself and another to other people?
- Have I got the facts right?
- Am I just tired and irritable?

4 Challenge your own perspective on the situation:
- Maybe there's been a mistake or I've misunderstood?
- Have I checked that there's no other reason for this situation?
- Have I explained myself clearly?
- What's this doing to my health?
- Maybe I've jumped to conclusions too quickly?
- Ruminating like this may be harming me.
- I will act when I'm calm and have thought about it clearly.

Mindfulness

When people ruminate they tend to revisit past injustices or go into the future and fantasize about revenge. So bringing your mind into the present moment can be a powerful strategy. Say to yourself, 'Be here now!' Another mindfulness technique is to focus your mind on your senses and become aware of what is around you: the sights, sounds, smells and textures.

Rumination time

This is a useful technique to follow if you find you can't stop ruminating.

1 Set aside a regular time each day for ruminating – about 15 to 20 minutes once a day, and no more: set an alarm clock. Pick a time when you are free of interruptions.
2 Pick a place to ruminate, somewhere that you don't associate with relaxation (not your bed, or favourite chair). Some people sit at the foot of the stairs or at a table, on an upright chair. This will be the only place you should ruminate.
3 On a piece of paper write down the negative thoughts, all the things that you are dwelling on.
4 Stop when time's up – remember, set an alarm clock.

5 If any negative thoughts come up during the day, write them down on a piece of paper, and then tell yourself to stop thinking about them until your allotted time.

You will begin to understand your anger if you accept that your emotions and feelings are neither good nor bad, but that they are actually messengers. Then you can ask yourself what they are trying to tell you. When you feel angry or experience emotions related to anger (upset, annoyance, frustration, resentment, being judge-mental), then ask yourself: Is my anger masking feelings of fear or loss? If so, then acknowledge those feelings. If not, ask yourself if it is your ideas and beliefs that are being violated. Try to revise these ideas by changing them to more flexible ones.

When the stress and anxiety aren't shifting

After exiting a traumatic relationship with a sociopath, and with sufficient support from friends and family, you might hope that it's possible to move straightforwardly through the stages of coming to terms with the situation, from initial trauma to acceptance. However, no one can predict the outcome of this recovery process. Even with the best intentions some people end up enduring persistent stress and anxiety – an experience similar to, if not the same as, post-traumatic stress disorder. (Because it has primarily been identified by observing survivors of a specific range of traumatic events such as combat and disaster, the term PTSD fails to capture the consequences of prolonged, repeated trauma such as instances when a person is unable to flee and is under the control of an abuser, as may exist in families where abuse is taking place.)

PTSD is a severe anxiety disorder that can develop after exposure to any event that results in psychological trauma. According to one expert on surviving trauma, Judith Herman, captivity that brings the targeted person into prolonged contact with the perpetrator of the abuse creates a special type of relationship. She defines this as one of coercive control. This is equally true when the individual is rendered captive by physical, economic, social and psychological means, as in the case of battered partners or spouses and abused children.[6]

PTSD itself arises due to deregulation of the fear system. Fear is a necessary emotion at times of danger, and like anger is followed by a stress response – fighting, freezing or fleeing. This survival system depends on our ability to appraise threats in order to initiate survival behaviour. Once the threat or trauma is over, the fear system normally calms down after a few days or weeks. In PTSD this system fails to reset to normal, keeping the sufferer hyper-alert, on the lookout in case the event happens again.[7] The disorder is characterized by involuntary, persistent remembering or reliving of the traumatic event in flashbacks, vivid memories and recurrent dreams. Usually this is accompanied by problems such as depression, substance abuse, and other anxiety disorders. The person may feel emotionally numb, for example feeling detached from others.

PTSD occurs when the trauma inflicted on an individual threatens her psychological integrity and overwhelms her ability to cope. As an effect of psychological trauma, PTSD is more enduring than the more commonly seen fight-or-flight response (also known as acute stress response), and is indicated by symptoms such as flashbacks, sleep problems, difficulty in concentrating, and being emotionally labile (moods go up and down: the person is elated one moment, miserable the next). Chronically traumatized people are often hyper-vigilant, anxious and agitated. Over time they may complain not only of insomnia, startle reactions and agitation, but also of numerous other physical symptoms. Tension headaches, gastrointestinal disturbances and abdominal, back or pelvic pain are extremely common. Individuals also frequently complain of tremors, choking sensations or nausea. Repeated trauma appears to intensify the physiological symptoms.

For a formal diagnosis of PTSD to be made, the symptoms should have lasted more than one month and be causing significant impairment in the person's social, occupational, or other important areas of functioning. When the symptoms are mild and have been present for less than four weeks after the traumatic events last occurred, the guidelines recommend keeping a watchful eye and waiting. But managing the chaos, material losses, grief and anger is down to the individual person, and how and when he or she regains control.

The clinical literature points to an association between bodily disorders and childhood trauma. Some survivors of prolonged childhood abuse develop severe dissociation, cutting themselves off and becoming detached from their feelings and other people. At the other extreme, one study conducted in 1989 described a process the researchers called 'mind-fragmenting operations, where abused children were deluded into thinking that their abusive parents were good parents'.[8]

Prolonged trauma at the hands of a sociopath may have emotional impacts, such as protracted depression. Here the chronic symptoms of PTSD combine with the symptoms of depression, producing what has been called the **survivor triad** of insomnia, nightmares and psychosomatic complaints. The humiliated rage of the traumatized person adds to the burden. He has been unable to express anger at his perpetrator: to do so would have jeopardized his survival. So even when released from the perpetrator's grip, he continues to be afraid of expressing his anger. Furthermore, the individual often carries a burden of unexpressed anger against all those who remained indifferent and failed to help. Efforts to control this rage may further exacerbate his social withdrawal and paralysis of initiative while occasional outbursts of rage against others may further alienate him and prevent the restoration of relationships. Internalization of rage may result in self-hatred, even thoughts of suicide. Even though major depression is frequently diagnosed in survivors of prolonged abuse, the connection with the preceding trauma is frequently lost. Hence patients are incompletely treated because the traumatic origins of the intractable depression have not been recognized.

Dealing with traumatic memories

Depression, severe anxiety and fear commonly stem from traumatic memories. People distressed by such memories may be constantly reliving them through nightmares or flashbacks, and may withdraw from their family or social circle in order to avoid exposing themselves to reminders of those memories. They may become physically aggressive, argumentative or moody, causing difficulties in relationships with their family, spouse or partner, and children. Sometimes they resort to substance abuse, drugs or alcohol in order to deal with the anxiety. If symptoms of apathy, impulsive behaviour, sleeplessness or irritability persist, the person may want to discuss this with his or her family doctor and to seek the help of a psychotherapist.

The management of traumatic memories is important when treating PTSD. Traumatic memories are stressful and can emotionally overwhelm a person's existing coping mechanisms. When simple objects such as a photograph, or events such as a birthday party, evoke traumatic memories, people often try to remove the unwanted memory from their minds in order to proceed with life, but this approach usually has only limited success. Over time the frequency of these triggers or memory joggers diminishes for most people, and for some the number of intrusive memories diminishes rapidly as the person adjusts to the situation. For others, however, they may continue for decades and interfere with the person's mental, physical and social well-being.

Several psychotherapies have been developed that weaken or prevent the formation of traumatic memories. Cognitive behavioural therapies have been found to be effective methods of reducing the emotional distress and negative thought patterns associated with traumatic memories in those with PTSD and depression. One such therapy is **trauma-focused therapy**. This involves bringing the traumatic memory or memories to mind and with the aid of a therapist restructuring the way the memories are thought about. Another is **eye movement desensitization and reprocessing** (EMDR). This involves elements of exposure therapy (where you systematically confront your fears) and cognitive behavioural therapy (which addresses unhelpful ways of thinking about your situation, and the things you do as a result), although there is still some debate as to whether it works. EMDR begins by identifying disturbing memories, cognitions and sensations. Then the negative thoughts are found that are associated with each memory. While both memory and thought are held in mind, the person follows a moving object with her eyes. Afterwards, a positive thought about the memory is discussed in an effort to replace the negative thought associated with the memory with a more positive thought.

Pharmacological methods for erasing traumatic memories are currently being researched, although this raises ethical concerns. The use of drugs to blunt the impact of traumatic memories treats human emotional reactions to life events as a medical issue, which may not necessarily be a good thing and may expose individuals to unnecessary risk. If drug treatments are administered unnecessarily – when for example a person could learn to cope without drugs – the person may needlessly be exposed to side effects. And the loss of painful memories may actually end up causing more harm than good. Painful, frightening or even traumatic memories can serve to teach us to avoid certain situations or experiences. By removing those memories their function in warning and protecting individuals may be lost.

Medication can sometimes be helpful following a trauma, but it is important for the person diagnosed with PTSD to see a medical doctor for regular check-ups. UK guidance from the National Institute for Health and Clinical Excellence (NICE) advises that drug treatments (paroxetine or mirtazapine for general use, amitriptyline or phenelzine for initiation only by mental health specialists) should be considered for the treatment of PTSD in adults who express a preference not to engage in trauma-focused psychological treatment. There have been significant advances in the medical treatment of PTSD; nevertheless, as is the case in other anxiety disorders, few long-term trials have been performed, and there is a lack of data on the effectiveness of treatment.

Individuals with PTSD can also become ill with depression. Depression can be treated either with antidepressant medication, or with talking treatments such as counselling or psychotherapy. It is important in such cases, when the symptoms ascribed to PTSD persist, to speak about them openly with someone and get professional help. The important message to take from all this is that by reaching out for support, seeking medical advice and treatment, and developing new coping skills, individuals can at the very least learn to manage effectively the symptoms of PTSD and better still, overcome the problem in time.

6

Establishing boundaries and regaining control of your life

Once you have shaken off the sociopath, dusted yourself down and regained some control over your life, there are decisions to be made about the longer term. In this chapter we will highlight the internal and external resources and know-how you will need to get back on track and guard yourself against further sociopathic abuse.

Coping in the aftermath of trauma

Re-establishing control after a one-off encounter

It is not sociopaths who change their behaviour; unfortunately they leave that responsibility to the rest of us. Sociopaths have no reason to modify their behaviour because the motivation and opportunities persist for them to carry on abusing other people.

In the case of a one-off brush with a sociopath, the chances are that all you need is to establish some boundaries to your relationship so you regain some control over the situation. For instance, if you work with a colleague who has sociopathic tendencies and you fear she will attempt to sabotage your work or damage your reputation in some way, keep a record of her correspondence, including emails, in order to regain control. Another way to reassert control is to restrict future communications. For instance, you could insist that all correspondence go through a third party; if the option is available, you might even avoid communicating with your abusive colleague altogether. It all depends upon your work circumstances, and the circumstances within which the sociopath operates. If the sociopath has some jurisdiction over you – as your boss or supervisor, for example – you may need to consider making a formal complaint of harassment.

Bullying and harassment

Bullying and harassment in the workplace should not be tolerated. Sexual harassment is one of the most common forms of harassment and in the UK is specifically outlawed by the Equality Act 2010. The Advisory, Conciliation and Arbitration Service (ACAS), an organization devoted to preventing and resolving employment disputes, argues that it is in the interest of the company you work for to make clear what sort of behaviour would be considered harassment and what would constitute bullying. **Harassment** is unwanted conduct which has the purpose or effect of violating an individual's dignity or creating an intimidating, hostile, degrading, humiliating or offensive environment for that individual. **Bullying** is most often characterized as offensive, intimidating, malicious or insulting behaviour, an abuse or misuse of power through means that undermine, humiliate, denigrate or injure the recipient.

It is good practice for employers to give examples of what is unacceptable behaviour in their company. This may include the following:

- spreading malicious rumours, or insulting someone (particularly on the grounds of age, race, sex, disability, sexual orientation and religion or belief);
- copying memos that are critical about someone to others who don't need to know;
- ridiculing or demeaning someone – picking on them or setting them up to fail;
- exclusion from a team, colleagues or a task;
- victimization;
- unfair treatment, such as being asked to do unnecessary tasks, or penalized without cause;
- overbearing supervision, or other misuse of power or position;
- unwelcome sexual advances – touching, standing too close, display of offensive materials, asking for sexual favours, making decisions on the basis of sexual advances being accepted or rejected;
- making threats or comments about job security without foundation;
- deliberately undermining a competent worker by overloading and constant criticism;

- preventing an individual progressing by intentionally blocking promotion or training opportunities.

If the bullying occurs in school, as in the case of James (our socio-path in Chapter 2) and Sam (the target), it is important as a parent or carer to communicate your concerns to the school at the earliest opportunity, and to work with the school to resolve the problem. Bullying is often exacerbated by the fact that some of the victim's peers don't want to lose status by associating with him, or are keen to avoid the risks of being bullied themselves, so increasing the isolation of the person on the receiving end. Since 1999, all UK schools have been legally required to have an anti-bullying policy. However, bullying is by nature an insidious problem. So if your child's behaviour suddenly changes, don't assume it is just related to hormones and puberty. Instead, talk to her; it could be indicative of something far more troubling.

If the sociopathic bully is a friend or neighbour, be vigilant and record any unusual goings-on. If you are experiencing harassment or intimidating behaviour yourself, don't ignore it – most of the time it is unlikely to go away without some kind of action. Don't feel it is your fault, or fear being labelled as a 'troublemaker' for bringing it to the attention of other people and the relevant author-ities. People who are involved in harassing behaviour often display it as a form of control and 'superiority' over your life; if you ignore it, this may be seen by the sociopath as a sign of success.

Even if you have only been harassed once, don't hesitate to contact someone for help. If the situation warrants it – if for instance your safety or someone else's is at risk, or property has been damaged – inform your local police and ask them for help. Ask them about the Protection from Harassment Act of 1997 (PFHA '97) and other legal avenues that might be open to you. The PFHA defines harassment as a 'course of conduct', meaning that for behaviour to amount to harassment it must occur on at least two occasions. Originally both occasions needed to involve the same person, but in 2005 the Act was amended by the Serious Organized Crime and Police Act so that 'pursuing a course of conduct' could mean approaching two people just once. Ask the police if they are able to take action on your behalf under the relevant legislation, and in particular the PFHA '97. Another option is to seek legal help from a solicitor.

You could also talk to a harassment adviser (you may have one in your workplace or company) or seek the help of a counsellor. Don't ever approach your neighbour or the person who is harassing you if you are in any way worried that there may be actual physical danger or that violence may be threatened. Call the police at once if this is the case. If you decide to approach the person responsible for harassing you, take due care over your safety. Do *not* go alone; take a friend or relative with you. Taking a witness will allow you to have a third-party account of what was said and done; the person harassing you cannot then claim that you didn't ask him to stop. Above all, your safety is paramount; do not place yourself in unnecessary danger.

Is it ever advisable to tell someone that they are sociopathic?

We don't advise you to confront someone with the notion that they are sociopathic, narcissistic or psychopathic, or for that matter borderline, even if you are absolutely certain they exhibit the traits. Even if the person concerned occasionally appears to be aware that she doesn't react like people around her, sociopaths rarely think badly of themselves. They don't have the same emotional attachment to ideas and concepts that 'normal' people do. However, she may know she is different. Being relatively unemotional, she can be fearless. Often sociopaths use this to their advantage, staying calm when others are afraid. Trying to make them feel remorse, guilt or shame is useless and can encourage them to fake feelings, to go along with the game.

Whether someone knows or is informed that they are sociopathic depends a lot upon their social and cultural background. But nowadays, with the advent of the internet and social media, it must be hard for sociopaths not to get wind of the concept of sociopathy or know something of the phenomenon. And their self-absorbed nature makes it highly likely that many of them have read widely on the issue and even diagnosed themselves.

Establishing control following prolonged contact with a sociopath

A full recovery from a traumatic encounter with a sociopath means recapturing your zeal for life. This requires a certain amount of self-growth. Getting over the experience is not always easy. It can be a battle, difficult and discouraging at times. The good news is that the vast majority of us get there in the end – but recovering from the experience often requires us to challenge the perspectives and rules that have sustained our belief systems and the belief systems of those around us. This can cause conflict before it brings us release or resolution, because often the way we live our life is something handed down to us from our parents and shaped by the culture we're immersed in.

A growing body of literature suggests that recovery is characterized by predictable stages and milestones (see Figure 2). Within each stage there are developmental tasks and skills to master, perspectives to develop and issues to address before moving to the next stage. Change not only comes about in recognizable stages but is more likely to happen when changing is important to us, and we are confident in pulling it off. If this makes it sound easy, we acknowledge that it isn't. Most of us tend not to go through change in a neat and linear fashion; in fact the direction of travel can be a little bit messy, with movement back and forth. Things begin to steady as you gain confidence in the process and thankfully, most of us get there in the end.

Change requires us to actively engage in the process. We have assets, both internal and external, collectively called **recovery capital**, which support us in dealing with changing circumstances. Every one of us possesses internal reserves of recovery capital that initiate and sustain our own recovery, but sometimes we need a little help in identifying what we've got. Sometimes to aid the process we also need a change in self-perception, or somehow to 'repair' our identity.

It can help to seek out others who have a shared goal. People recovering from a traumatic relationship with a sociopath often find recovery-supportive friendships beneficial. Such friendships need to be natural (reciprocal), accessible to you at times of greatest need, and potentially enduring. It can also make a real difference if a positive person is around to witness your change. In her book *Banished Knowledge: Facing Childhood Injuries*, the author and child abuse expert Alice Miller identified this sort of person as an 'enlightened witness'; someone willing to support a harmed individual and help him gain understanding of his past experiences.

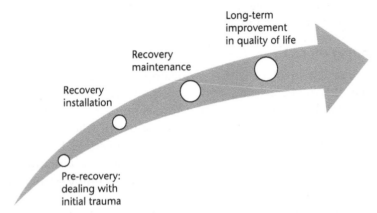

Figure 2   The recovery process

In this context an enlightened witness is anyone who is insightful and empathetic enough to help you face up to your difficulties and regain your autonomy. If you are isolated and no such witness is immediately available, social media and the internet can prove a helpful route to support. The change process is often messy, so if you become engaged in peer support you may find yourself flitting between roles, from acting helpless to engaging in the act of helping others. This is entirely normal and healthy given the tentative nature of the recovery process.

Coping day to day

Establishing personal boundaries

It is important after you have experienced a trauma involving a sociopath to re-establish your personal boundaries. One of the best moves you can make is to introduce and reinforce new rules of engagement. This may or may not include a rule of 'no contact'. A rule of no contact is easier said than implemented, but can be very necessary in order to prevent further trauma. The move is a lot easier to carry off if at the final showdown the sociopath walks out of your life; nevertheless, *you* may have to initiate the rule and take affirmative action yourself. The right approach – whether merely to limit contact or to apply a no-contact rule – depends on your individual circumstances, but whatever route you take, stay alert to the sociopath's persistent games and stand firm; sociopaths have a tendency to draw you in again.

Limiting contact

Many people involved with a sociopath limit contact at the point when the drama reaches critical pitch. Each person's situation is unique, however, and it is best to determine for yourself what contact you are prepared to accept. For a parent whose partner is a sociopath, this is an especially difficult, stressful and confusing time. Not only are you dealing with the trauma of a destructive relationship, you are working out how to handle future relations in order to protect your children.

It is not uncommon for a sociopath to behave badly and in an extreme fashion as soon as he realizes you want to reduce or stop contact. He may become disruptive and manipulative in an attempt to regain control. On the plus side, most give up hassling and manipulating you eventually; usually when they set their sights on a new target. Nevertheless, limiting contact with a sociopath requires you to be firm. You have to learn to assert yourself and your needs, which will help you in your own recovery.

That said, if you think the sociopath is potentially dangerous, and you perceive that you, some other adult or any children are still at risk, you should seek help from the authorities: the police, social services and legal advisers. Another important piece of advice is to keep written records of all agreements and discussions involving adults at risk of harm, and agreements about the welfare of children. Keep all written statements in a safe place, as you will need ample evidence if you decide to take legal action at a later date.

No contact

In most other circumstances it is probably best to have no contact at all with a person you identify as a sociopath. While it can be quite straightforward to cut ties with someone who is relatively new in your life, if the sociopath is part of your social group or family, a friend or partner of long standing, it becomes more complicated. You should ensure that other friends and acquaintances know you are no longer in contact with the individual concerned, and ask them not to play 'go-between'. You will also need to make it clear that you don't want to discuss anything about the socio-pathic person (or people). Refuse to accept information from a third party and if people try to involve you, tell them not to involve themselves in this way as it could damage relations between you.

The leaking of communication to and from third parties is the most common mistake people make following the establishment of a no-contact rule. Although it may be natural curiosity on your part to hear the third party out, it can reopen wounds to hear what the sociopath is saying about you or doing in her life, so stop people immediately if they begin telling you anything, and let them know you are not prepared to hear or say anything about the person who has abused you. If the third party refuses to respect your wishes, you should consider limiting contact with him or her as well.

For those whose lives have been heavily intermeshed with one or more sociopaths, in a family for instance, a no-contact rule can be extremely hard to apply. You will have to decide who to cut out completely, as well as what to do about communication with family members on the periphery of the situation. Again, you may have to spell out the boundaries to avoid further conflict.

Cutting ties is a painful and terminal step but typically a nec-essary one. On the upside, it is a significant step on the road to recovery. One way of doing it is to write a frank letter stating that the relationship is over and you don't wish to be contacted again. A phone call or email seems easy, but can lead to the mistake of getting into continued dialogue and bartering. Once a no-contact rule is set, there are things you need to iron out. Do you remove phone messages without listening to them? Block the person on Facebook and Twitter? Do you accept apologies? Gifts?

If messages are left on an answering machine, or you receive emails or calls from the person concerned, you must resist the temptation to respond. If the person catches you unaware and you pick up a call, hang up immediately. Call blocking is another option, and is inexpensive. Sociopaths like playing games with your emotions, and having access to you after a relationship is over is like letting the game continue. If your sociopath does harass you in this way, keep all his communications in case you decide to pursue a harassment charge at some later stage, as this is potential evidence. If you wish to save the evidence but think you would be too tempted to read it or to act on the contents, immediately give any communiqués to a trusted third party or to a solicitor, who can keep them stored away safely with your other important personal effects. It is probably advisable to block or change your email. If anything gets through, delete it as soon as you recognize the sender without opening or reading it (the exception to the rule being if you feel you need it as evidence). Do not get into games with the sociopath by entering into dialogue again.

Preventing lapses in judgement

Having an enlightened witness around will help to keep the person in recovery on the right path. It is not uncommon to feel isolated in the early days once you are removed from immediate danger, perhaps in completely new surroundings. After the initial relief has worn off, you may feel disorientated, ambivalent and lonely. Feeling alone is quite a normal response to change and unfamiliar circumstances, and it's one that the sociopath will play on, angered by your snub and the change you have made in the rules of engagement. Often at this point a sociopath will accelerate his games. He may make you question your sanity, your perception of what happened, everything and everyone you hold dear. He may even feign remorse to try to win you back, a response that is hard to ignore if you are feeling lonely and excluded.

Meanwhile others who don't know the full extent of your situation may make judgements and disparaging remarks, particularly if you have left a marriage, job or family. This sort of reaction sadly comes with the territory, as those who make a stand are often harshly judged by others who are uninformed and look on with untrained eyes. And let us not forget that most of those who criticize you are likely to belong to the 60 per cent of apaths that make up the majority, many of whom may fear your newfound voice and strength. If this happens, just remember it is most likely your freedom of spirit and nonconformity that triggers social anxiety, rather than there being anything discernibly wrong with you. This is why it is important not to withdraw and become isolated at such a critical moment. Instead, the best route out of the situation is to keep good people (including those enlightened witnesses) about you and let them buoy you up until you are confident in your unconventionality and accept it as one of your strengths.

For all your good intentions about maintaining limited contact, or breaking it altogether, sometimes we trip up. There will be situations to look out for and set-ups to avoid until new behaviours and habits are bedded down and become the norm. In the intervening period you need to learn how not to set yourself up and become entangled again in the sociopath's life. In some ways, weaning someone off a destructive relationship is like weaning them from an addictive substance or behaviour. In both situations the relationship and pattern of behaviour are often deeply entrenched. It takes time to gain confidence in our ability to make what are sometimes sweeping life changes, and time to adopt new sets of behaviour. It takes patience and a willingness to learn from trial and error to sustain changes and fully adapt. But one advantage the non-sociopathic in society have over the sociopathic is the ability to change. The sociopath is unable to do this; his or her persona is fixed. The sociopath lacks the insight and the ability to learn from his or her mistakes. In addition the sociopath's behaviour is fairly predictable. In essence sociopaths behave the way they do because they are motivated by a need for stimulus and seek out opportunities to take advantage of. Figure 3 sums this up diagrammatically.

Once you take this on board, it is up to you to identify ways to block opportunities for the sociopath to snare you again. Using the straightforward approach outlined overleaf, it is possible to identify cues and triggers to avoid relapsing into old ways and back into relations with the sociopath. Becoming more aware of our former ways and behaviours helps us gain insight, which helps prevent us inadvertently getting trapped in a cycle of sociopathic abuse.

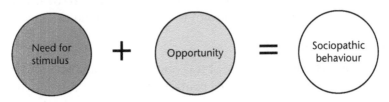

Figure 3   Motivators for sociopathic behaviour

Stop making seemingly irrelevant decisions (SIDs)

A seemingly irrelevant decision, or SID, is a decision or choice that may appear unimportant or insignificant on the surface but actually increases the likelihood that the person making it will be placed in a high-risk situation that can cause a relapse to his or her former behaviour. A person may ignore, deny or explain away the importance of these decisions and choices. The identification of SIDs is an important part of the relapse prevention treatment first devised by psychologists G. Alan Marlatt and J. R. Gordon and used with people with addictive behaviours. We think it is a useful approach for weaning yourself off old behaviours that result in you succumbing to the sociopath's ploys.

Examples of SIDs include:

- driving past the sociopath's home on your way back from work;
- idly 'Googling' the sociopath or checking her Facebook page;
- asking after the sociopath to third parties who are still in contact with her;
- finding some reason to send the sociopath an email;
- texting the sociopath on her birthday or some other special occasion.

All these are seemingly innocuous, but can put you in the path of danger. Perhaps, as you drive past the sociopath's house, she sees you drive by and waves. That one small act gives her licence to call you and you become hooked in again. Perhaps checking the sociopath's Facebook page makes you feel sad and you begin reminiscing – before you know it you have sent her a personal message. Curiosity is not a bad thing; it is natural in many circumstances. It is an emotion related to natural inquisitive behaviour and connected to learning. But in this situation we need to recognize its disastrous consequences and learn to control the impulse.

The rule violation effect

This effect is evident when we break our own rules and boundaries. It can apply to either a limited contact or no-contact rule that has been set in place. The rule violation effect (RVE) refers to the tendency of an individual, having made a personal commitment not to contact the sociopath, to revert to uncontrolled contact following a single lapse. The RVE comes into play when the person attributes the cause of the initial lapse to internal factors within himself, such as a lack of willpower or believing himself to be missing the socio-path (or rather, the person he *believed* the sociopath to be).

With these lapse and relapse prevention strategies the aim is to learn how to minimize the risk of relapse (i.e. prevent the RVE) by directing attention to the more controllable external or situational factors that triggered the lapse (e.g. high-risk situations, coping skills and anticipated outcomes), so that you can quickly return to the goal of no contact and not 'lose control' (i.e. get back in contact). Specific intervention strategies may help you identify and cope with high-risk situations and manage lapses. These are considered next.

High-risk situations

Moods

You may have low moods, bad moods, increased anxiety or irri-tability when you break off contact. These are temporary feelings and will get easier over time. You may over-react to things that nor-mally wouldn't bother you. This is common. Try to find new ways of coping with emotions like anger, upset, annoyance and stress. These tips may help you:

- Discover new ways of dealing with negative feelings rather than ruminating on the past.
- Remind yourself that the feeling is temporary; it will go away.
- Congratulate yourself for coping with life without the sociopath.
- Ask others to understand and be patient.
- Do things that make you feel good.
- Try to get a good night's sleep, and if having trouble sleeping, seek advice about improving your chances of sleeping well.

If you get good or bad news that affects your mood, dwelling on the past or seeking out the sociopath will not change the news, whether good or bad, or help the situation. It will only reduce your chances of changing your situation. Have a good cry; tell someone how you are feeling. Take slow deep breaths over a period of a few minutes to help you relax.

Habits and routines

You may have developed certain habits and routines in your life with the sociopath. It's therefore important to consider changing your routine so you don't experience cues and triggers about him; that's a situation that can lead you to take SIDs, to lapse or end up violating newly established rules.

Just as a reminder, here are our tips again for coping with stress:

- Work it off by taking a walk in the fresh air.
- Talk to someone you really trust.
- Learn to accept what you cannot change.
- Don't self-medicate with alcohol, too much coffee or tranquillizers.
- Get enough sleep and rest.
- Take time out for activities you really enjoy, or try out some fresh ones such as new forms of exercise, doing something creative or picking up a different hobby.
- Doing something for others can make you feel good too.
- Take one thing at a time.
- Prioritize your day ahead and only do the things you have to do.
- Don't be afraid to say 'no'.
- Eating good meals at regular times will help your mood.
- Know when you are tired and do something about it.
- Be realistic about what you can achieve. Forget perfection.

Triggers

A trigger is something that you associate with something or someone else, and to which you are likely to respond. Years of conditioning from a sociopath mean that a particular trigger will set off a reaction in you by a process of association, much as a dog can be conditioned to respond to a ringing bell in the same way as to food. Here we introduce and adapt some ideas of psychologist B. J. Fogg, who refers to triggers as phenomena that are either 'hot' or 'cold'. A **hot trigger** is something that affects you immediately: someone yelling at you or demanding something of you, or being stuck in a traffic jam. A **cold trigger** is something that affects you indirectly: the sociopath's double or doppelganger on television or in an advert, or a letter with familiar-looking handwriting. A hot trigger forces an immediate response, while the effects of a cold trigger build up over time. Triggers work as a call to action and can cause us to act on impulse. To avoid lapsing into previous behaviour it helps to find a way to disconnect our feelings from the object of association. The steps to breaking the connections involve:

Looking for patterns First we need to see clearly the things that make us think about the sociopath and other people we have removed from our lives or have lost as a result of changing our behaviour. Once we recognize the kind of things that work as hot or cold triggers – the sort that trigger an unhelpful reaction in us – it is useful to a make a mental note of them.

Becoming more 'trigger-savvy' Give yourself a chance to analyse your own triggers and see if you can devise ways to break the associations. Maybe just being cognisant of the fact that a trigger can arouse unwanted feelings and memories is enough. Maybe you need to talk yourself out of reacting whenever a trigger arrives uninvited. Understanding how best to dampen the effects of emerging triggers is necessary in driving behaviour change forward. Here's an example.

Jill
Jill had not been in contact with her sociopathic father for several months when a message from him appeared in her email box one afternoon. She immediately recognized this as a trigger, and knew that if she opened and responded to the email she would be in a high risk situation, in jeopardy of responding and thus lapsing. Because she was mindful of this situation arising, she recognized the position she was in and instead of responding on impulse, as she previously might have done, she calmly deleted the message and got back on with finishing her report, avoiding the high risk situation.

How other people coped

Let's see now, in their own words, how some of the many survivors of sociopathic abuse have managed to deal with the trauma. Some individuals' names have been changed to protect their identities.

Nancy Ellen Iandoli
Years of counselling gave me the tools to learn to set boundaries with my narcissistic mother and my sociopathic adult son (my father is deceased, I am an only child). I have been fortunate to have found quality counsellors who utilized the EMDR method in their sessions. I learned to grieve for the loss of my dream to have both a loving mother and a loving son. I stopped engaging in any communication with both of them. I owe my life to my two wonderful counsellors, Larry and Joyce; they helped me deal with my rage and disappointment. They helped me to develop the courage to move forward with my life.

I learned to accept what I cannot change, but that does not mean I like it, I will always have post-traumatic stress disorder. The depth of the loss and betrayal of the two people who should be the closest to me has been heart wrenching. There is no getting over the pain, but the anguish diminishes over time. Support groups on the internet have led me to other survivors – their validation and support is very healing and soothing, and I am able to help others too.

Colleen Fourie

As a child I lived in my head a lot; I escaped into fantasy and daydreams and books. What really saved me was the birth of my first daughter . . . That awakened in me a powerful instinct to protect and to survive. She was my first true love, the first clean, beautiful, shining soul in a sordid cynical world. For the first time I was able to feel what was right and what was wrong, and gradually it started dawning on me that I was not the 'bad one', but the one who had been wronged . . . It is still dawning. I'm not there yet.

Paul

My therapy was focused as much on my mother as it was on my marriage. I believed my mother was perfect. Actually it verged on mother worship. She was never wrong, she knew what I needed to do with my life; my school major was her choice, my job was her choice. At times I felt as if my mother was omniscient and all-knowing, weird as that sounds. At 28, I broke this mould and began making more of my own choices. My entire family came down against it. I stayed away from Mom and began to grow a little. My dad seemed to have a midlife crisis when I reached puberty. He changed and became a cruel and selfish person and rejected me after that.

My earlier counselling was focused on recognizing my emotions. I had learned as a child to ignore them. All emotions were against my mother's religion; love = lust = bad and anger = rebellion = bad. As my therapy progressed I healed and my emotions thawed out. When my ex-wife cheated on me I got depressed and told her. She denied that I was. 'No you are not,' she would say, but I knew I was as I had begun to contemplate suicide. But then I realized that that was a permanent solution to a temporary problem. I then remembered my earlier therapy and let myself feel, and began to get angry.

My ex-wife was a serial cheater and there were many times when she behaved strangely and I just justified it to myself. But after the divorce these would reappear to me and a new understanding emerged. Finally I was able to see her as a flawed human like myself. This didn't mean I contacted her or gave her the grace to heal, because she is on her own journey and probably wouldn't understand. What little contact I have with her has convinced me she is still a narcissist and would take my overtures the wrong way. My current wife is very strong and understands my weaknesses and strengths; we have a serenity that we will not give up for any amount of material comforts or gold.

Lizzie

I was an anxious child, a worrier. As I grew up I came to appreciate that my sister was 'different'. She could be charming, but she had a cold, callous streak. No one else seemed to notice and I felt very afraid and alone with my concerns. My mother is also sociopathic, though obviously as a child I had no idea. Most of my mother's unpleasant behaviour was directed at people outside the family. At home she was the matriarch whom we all obeyed. I was a little scared of her and feared her rejection. I know I consciously strove to please her, but she was very critical of me.

I finally started to find my own voice in my twenties. It was then that my relations with the family soured. My mother turned very nasty. I think she sensed she was losing control over me. It wasn't until my forties that I began to realize that I couldn't cope any more – I couldn't take their abuses any longer and got away. Leaving the family, stopping contact, was a very traumatizing experience. What has helped me more than anything is having a supportive and loving husband and a wonderful son. I am still wary of other people and trust is a big issue for me. Coming from a family where sociopathy is rife is very stigmatizing. I rarely tell anyone about it. Recently I joined an online group and I've met others there with similar experiences. That has helped relieve me of some of the burden – finally I have somewhere I can offload the guilt and shame. I still feel unnatural for exiting the family in this way. I feel people judge me for it. But it was the right thing to do for my sanity's sake.

Debrieanna

I thought I'd met my Prince Charming and I was living in a fairy tale. In reality, I *was* living a fairy tale . . . his. His reality, what he pretended to be, was a lie. A deceptive mask of his choosing for each person he used, abused and discarded. The end always justified the means; I was just one of his toys.

Lies, deceit, manipulation. The red flags were there, I chose not to see them. He gaslighted me into believing I was sick, not him. The fairy tale became a nightmare. When he finally left, after planning it for two years, it got worse. He became nasty and cruel. For him, it was a game to win. He couldn't break me, but I lost all trust in everyone, including myself.

How did I get through this? Lots of prayer. My faith and trust in God along with family and friends' emotional support. That got me through it. Good eventually overcame the evil. My life went from his darkness into my Light.

Bryan Stuart

I am a confident person now but I haven't always been. I have had major knockbacks in my life, but the way I deal with problems is by talking to those I love most. My story is that I had a run-in with my grandmother, the last person you would imagine. She seemed nice on the surface, but used to make odd remarks to me when the two of us were alone. For example, when I was about five years old she came up to me and said, 'Your father doesn't love you or your mum.' She made me think my father was going to leave us, when in actual fact this was far from true; my parents were happy together.

When you are five years old this is upsetting to hear. My grand-mother told me these lies on and off for several years. I was so disturbed by them that it affected my behaviour. I couldn't sleep at night and felt anxious all the time. Eventually, I told my parents, who were aghast. They weren't angry with me, but they were angry with my grand-mother, and rightly so! I have no idea to this day why she picked on me in this way.

We didn't have contact with my grandmother for some time after that, but because my parents thought it wasn't fair on me not to see my grandparents they eventually agreed for me to see them for a brief visit. I was about nine years old by this time. The visit escalated into one of the most horrific and scary days of my life. My grandmother must have been angry with me for telling my parents, and I think she wanted to get back at me. When my grandfather was out of the room she told me awful things about my parents, and other stuff meant for adult ears, disgusting things. She was also very rough with me physically and shoved me around. When I got home I told my parents the visit had gone well, because I was a bit scared and ashamed and doubted it had happened. I doubted myself!

After the ordeal we went on holiday but I just couldn't hold it in any more. I broke down and told my parents everything. Of course it was hard for me to tell them all the things my grandmother had said, but I felt a lot better knowing I had told them. They helped me so much then, and comforted me. Afterwards, I felt like I had made it all up, even though deep down I knew that I hadn't. But it was all so absurd. Telling others of my ordeal reassured me and brought me to my senses.

This major setback was something I wasted countless days and months worrying about. After finding the guts to talk about my ordeal to people I trust I've never looked back. I wish I'd had a book like this when I was going through it because there's no help or advice about getting over it. The best thing was speaking up and having people around who believed me and supported me.

Ian Carter

From early adolescence onwards I was always seen as the black sheep of the family. No one told me why. I went from a straight 'A' student to a punk. I thought I was rebelling but in fact I was responding to a sociopathic mother and an apathetic father.

From adolescence I had hated my father for being aggressive and angry all the time and my mother for being weak and the victim. What I was not aware of at the time was how the situation was being played out and manipulated by my mother. I now recognize my mother was the person with the problem, but it didn't seem so back then. She was so good at seeking pity and playing the victim. Yet in reality she was in control of the situation, and had to be the centre of attention.

When I was very young she used to dress me up in white suits (this *was* the early seventies!). I couldn't play with friends in case I got the clothes dirty. She would rather show me off to her friends as if I was a prized object. She never showed me affection, not even in private.

Our father used to sleep during the day as he often worked night shifts. Our mother would tell me and my siblings not to talk loudly during the day in case it angered our father. As a consequence we became very afraid of him. All through my growing up my mother would say we had no money, yet she was known for her extravagant dress and expensive tastes. In fact I remember her parading around in an expensive fur coat. Everything had to revolve around my mother and her wants. She controlled all aspects of family life, even though she acted hard done by.

My brother, my sister and I were pawns in a horrible game between my parents. After many heated rows between them, my father one day decided he had had enough of the situation. But instead of focusing his anger on my mother, he focused it on me. I admit that at 15 I was reacting against them. I no longer did everything the way my parents wanted and became less compliant, but I was not particularly wayward, quite the contrary: I was becoming increasingly withdrawn. In the end, my father told my mother she had to choose between him and me. She chose him. As a result, I was sent to live with my grandmother until I had finished my school exams.

Over the following two years I had periods of great instability. At one point I was destitute, homeless and had to claim state benefits to buy food. I was allowed occasional contact with my family but this was controlled by my mother, who always warned me not to upset my father, brother and sister. She continued to insist that I was the problem. Later I used my appearance as an act of rebellion. I became a punk! I looked aggressive but underneath I was still a quiet and peaceable character. Then at 19 I started my career. I wanted to help other people who might have experienced similar problems to me. I moved to another city and trained as a psychiatric nurse. Other people's problems seemed, in general, a lot simpler than my own.

I am now 42 years old and a company director, with a lovely wife and son. I am happy to say I am through the worst of the traumas caused by my sociopathic mother through my early childhood. Nevertheless I've had to stop all contact with my mother, brother and sister because they still view me as the problem and they were treating me and my family badly.

What has helped me? Being able to share and reflect on my thoughts with people that I love and who understand me. All of this has been really tough, especially having to break contact with family members and come to terms with the fact that my mother's influence has such great sway. I doubt my siblings will ever see me as I am, a decent and loving person. If I were to have contact with them it would just open up old wounds. This step to remove all contact has been very tough, but it's been worth it in the sense that I've got my self-respect back!

These words from survivors show us how the process of recovery is a transitional one. Recovery is about building a meaningful life as defined by the person him- or herself. In Chapter 7 we'll focus on the issues that arise when cutting ties or limiting contact with sociopaths who have been shielded within the family.

7

Dealing with complex family situations

Coping with the fallout

After separating from a sociopath you might think that things are finally sorted, but the sociopath is unlikely to cooperate as far as family responsibilities go. In fact, he is far more likely to try to turn things to his own advantage. Sadly, sociopaths' attentions often turn to their children, and not in a good way. They will frequently use their children as both shield and arsenal against you, the other parent.

This poses serious problems for the non-sociopathic parent and the ongoing welfare of his or her children. At an international level, the Convention on the Rights of the Child emphasizes the need to allow children a voice in any proceedings affecting their welfare. However, sociopaths are extremely good at manipulating others, including their own children, and will not hesitate to use them in a game of tug of war and attempt to alienate the non-sociopathic parent. This is exasperating enough when the sociopathic parent is the father, but even more so if it is the mother. This is because, thanks to the stereotype that a mother is always the better qualified person to care for younger children, the most common legal outcome of cases involving the care of children is that custody is awarded to the mother. As a result of this perception, the access rights of perfectly capable men can be denied in favour of women, even mothers who have demonstrated a poor track record of care.

When this applies to a sociopathic mother, it is a grave situation indeed. Largely because of this general legal stance, a new political trend, represented by fathers' rights and men's rights movements, has developed in recent years demanding equal parenting. Under this system there would be no legal determination of custody, and the rights of both parents to equal time with their child or children would be protected. In the USA, groups like Fathers 4

Justice (F4J), the American Coalition for Fathers and Children (ACFC), the Alliance for Non-Custodial Parents Rights (ANCPR), the Separated Parents Access & Resource Center (SPARC) and the National Congress for Fathers and Children (NCFC) are working on this nationally and internationally, and in the UK a similar move has emerged with groups like Parents 4 Protest and Fathers 4 Justice.

It is hard to accept this uncomfortable truth, but sociopaths don't love their children for themselves. Instead they view them as objects of manipulation. A non-sociopathic parent can thus be dealt a double blow at the hands of his or her former partner, and experience secondary trauma (a common term for the stress resulting from helping or wanting to help a traumatized or suffering person) whenever children or other loved ones are involved. There is internet support (see 'Useful addresses') for those facing the multifarious issues involved in coping as the partner of a sociopathic parent.

Being the partner of a sociopathic parent is like living on a minefield. On the whole sociopaths make poor parents. At best, they view their children as prized possessions. At worst, they actively try to corrupt them. In his book *Without Conscience*, Robert Hare states that sociopaths see children as an inconvenience. This indifference to their welfare takes many forms. They may leave young children alone or in the care of unreliable babysitters, or fail to provide them with proper food and clothing. They may demand certain behaviour or accomplishments for their own benefit. They may inflict physical and emotional abuse, or deliberately try to corrupt a child through inappropriate or dangerous activities. So when a sociopath is involved with children, always be on guard.

In light of this, the less interaction a sociopath has with his or her children the better, however harsh and unnatural this seems. If the non-sociopathic parent has instigated a limited or no-contact rule with the sociopathic parent, then the non-sociopathic parent can provide some counterbalance in the children's lives by offering genuine love, boundaries, nurturing and guidance. Children can and do cope remarkably well if they sense they are loved and feel safe, but this is hard to achieve when a sociopathic parent is present and stirring up perpetual conflict.

Many children eventually sense that there is no real bond between them and the sociopathic parent but it is, and will continue to be, a confusing and disturbing relationship for them. A good plan of action is to stay neutral whenever possible and say little about the sociopathic parent. Also, it is important to set boundaries in order to avoid children growing up thinking that sociopathic behaviour is acceptable. Over time you may learn to handle the new arrangement and situation effectively, like this father:

> My strategy now is not to give an inch on anything [with regard to the children], because she will take every possible opportunity to emotionally or otherwise manipulate every situation. You have to mean business and not get into a discussion or negotiation about anything. Zero tolerance is, unfortunately, the only approach that works for me.

Do not accept into your life anything or anyone that you don't want your children exposed to. Sociopathic family members and their apath 'friends' will have an impact on your children whether you realize it or not. So take steps to become assertive and more self-reliant. Arrange things as far as possible so that you are financially as well as socially independent of the sociopath who was formerly part of your life, otherwise you are allowing him control over you.

To compound the situation further, children may be brainwashed by their sociopathic parent into believing that the non-sociopathic parent is the problem and the root cause of the family's difficulties. The sociopathic parent may have only limited contact with her children, but it is important not to badmouth her even if you feel she deserves it. This is important for two reasons. First is the emotional well-being of the children, who should not feel trapped in the middle of the parents' issues with each other. Second, you need to avoid being accused of attempting parental alienation.

Parental Alienation Syndrome

In the UK and other countries such as the USA there is increasing recognition of Parental Alienation Syndrome (PAS). Although we feel some antipathy towards the move in recent years to medicalize so many aspects of human behaviour and everyday life, this response to children is unquestionably characteristic of the sociopath. It is an alienating tactic often employed by the sociopathic parent while simultaneously accusing the non-sociopathic parent of adopting it; thus he pulls off yet another gaslighting manoeuvre. PAS is understood as the systematic denigration by one parent of the other with the intent of alienating the child from the denigrated parent. The purpose of the alienation is usually to gain or retain sole custody, and it usually extends to the parent's family and friends as well. It is thought that a sociopathic mother is more likely to use this ploy against a non-sociopathic father, but it happens the other way round as well.

In his book *The Parental Alienation Syndrome*, Richard Gardner states that many children in this situation proudly declare their decision to reject the non-alienating parent as their own.[1] The children deny any contribution from their other parent, and the alienating parent often supports this. In fact, the alienating parent will often state that she wants the child to visit the other parent and will recognize the importance of such involvement, while indicating otherwise by her actions. Such children appreciate that, by stating the decision is their own, they mitigate the alienating parent's guilt and protect her from criticism. Their actions often earn these children praise from the alienating parent for being people with minds of their own, being brave enough to express their own opinions. Frequently, an alienating parent will press her children to tell her the truth regarding whether or not they really want to see their other parent. The children will often resort to saying that they hate the other parent and don't want to see him ever again.

If all this sounds depressing, remember that children usually work things out for themselves, so have faith. At some point they will realize that the sociopath cares only about him- or herself without you having to tell them and unintentionally pushing them away in the process. Nevertheless the systematic training and grooming of children in this way causes immense harm and damage to all sides. Many individuals who have gone through this experience say they didn't come to see what was going on until many years later, by which time a lot of damage had been caused to the individual and to family relations.

For children with one or more sociopathic parents it often takes years to come to terms with or understand their situation. Some never come to terms with it, or 'see' the reality of their circumstances. Indeed, in our experience it is not uncommon for children of sociopaths to reach a certain level of maturity, perhaps middle age, before they gain any proper understanding of their experiences. This is possibly because childhood experiences of this kind are so overwhelming that there is a tendency to block the painful memories until we are more capable of facing up to the trauma of early life.

Child protection

A child seldom needs a good talking to as a good listening to.

(Robert Brault, contemporary US freelance writer)

Within the domestic sphere, a particular family member, often a child, is sometimes targeted by his or her sociopathic kin. This may not come to light until the child is grown up and ready to face her past, but it is conceivable that she might approach a family member whom she trusts and try to unburden herself about the abuse that is going on. In such situations it is immensely important that the child is properly listened to and commended for speaking out. The uncomfortable truth, however, is that adults don't always accept that abuse is going on, especially if the abuser is a close family member. Hence children often learn to keep the abuse and their fears to themselves for fear of being rejected or told they are telling lies.

In her powerful book *The Body Never Lies*, Alice Miller notes that the parent or primary carer is to blame for any damage he inflicts upon his child, and must take full responsibility for participation in the abuse. Sociopaths don't own or take responsibility for the abuse they inflict upon others, but they must be held responsible all the same. And if other adults are involved in some way, albeit in not acting on an accusation of abuse or failing to 'see' the abuse, they must be held accountable for their inaction and negligence. Everyone who turns a blind eye to abuse of a child is, to some extent, blameworthy.

Let's recall the Sociopath-Empath-Apath Triad identified in Chapter 4. For sociopathic abuse to occur it usually requires the following threesome: the sociopath, the empath and the apath. As a reminder, the set-up goes like this:

- The empath is forced to make a stand on seeing the sociopath say or do something underhand.
- He challenges the sociopath, who throws others off the scent and blames the empath.

- The empath becomes an object of abuse when the apath corroborates the sociopath's side of the story.

If the empath is a child, and she comes forward and tells another family member or friend, a neighbour, aunt or uncle, and that adult does nothing to help the child, then this behaviour is morally inept; the kind of behaviour that is usually the preserve of the apath. It means the sociopath is likely to get away with enduring mistreatment of the child, while the child is likely to be at even greater risk of abuse now the sociopath knows she is a threat and capable of making a stand. In such circumstances, it may not be in the best interests of the child to remain in the family environment. However, sociopathic abuse of this kind, especially emotional abuse, rarely comes to the attention of the authorities and remains hidden, leaving the child unprotected and unsafe.

Child welfare – what to do if you suspect problems

Different countries have different laws governing the protection and safeguarding of children, but in the UK there is a comprehensive child welfare system under which local authorities have duties and responsibilities towards children in need in their area. This covers the provision of advice and services, accommodation and care of children who become uncared for, and also the capacity to initiate proceedings for the removal of children from their parents' care. Risk of 'significant harm' to children covers physical, sexual and emotional abuse and neglect. The basic legal principle in the UK, under the Children Act 1989, is that the welfare of the child is paramount.

Emotional abuse can affect a child from infancy, through adolescence, and into adulthood. It sets back a child's physical as well as mental development (the child's intelligence and memory) and puts a child at greater risk of developing mental health problems such as eating disorders and self-harming. It can also hamper a child's emotional development, including the ability to feel and express a full range of emotions appropriately or control his or her emotions. It can put children at greater risk of developing behavioural problems such as learning difficulties, problems with relationships and socializing, rebellious behaviour, aggressive and violent behaviour, anti-social behaviour and criminality and negative impulsive behaviour (not caring what happens to them). In the UK, the National Society for the

Children need to feel wanted, loved and safe; they also need consistency and boundaries. No parent or carer gets it right every time, and everyone has a bad day with their children, but emotional or physical abuse is different. Severe and persistent ill-treatment undermines a child's confidence and self-worth. Trauma survival specialist Judith Herman argues that as long as the target (in this case the child) maintains strong relationships with others, the perpetrator's power is limited; therefore, the sociopath seeks to isolate the child. The sociopath will not only attempt to prohibit communication and material support, but will also try to destroy the child's emotional ties to others. When the child is isolated, he increasingly becomes dependent on the sociopath, not only for survival and basic needs but for emotional sustenance. Prolonged confinement in fear and isolation reliably produces a bond of identification

Prevention of Cruelty to Children (NSPCC) suggests emotionally abusive behaviour includes:

- not responding to a child's emotional needs by persistently ignoring the child or being absent;
- humiliating or criticizing a child;
- disciplining a child with degrading punishments;
- not recognizing a child's individuality and limitations, pushing the child too hard, or being too controlling;
- exposing a child to distressing events or interactions, like domestic abuse or substance misuse;
- failing to promote a child's social development, for instance by not allowing the child to have friends.

You may notice a child and its parent have a difficult relationship. If the relationship is nervous, fearful or distant, or if you think the child's emotions, mental capacities or behaviour seem very different from other children of the same age, this may indicate a problem. If as an adult you do have valid concerns about a child being emotionally or physically abused, you should take action by contacting your local social services or police. Emotional abuse especially is often overlooked, yet the scars take longer to heal than any physical ones. Sadly, emotional abuse is far too common and is experienced daily by many children throughout the world. It is important to stop abuse in its tracks or better, prevent it entirely.

between the sociopath and the victim. This is another form of traumatic bonding and may occur between a battered partner and her abuser or between an abused child and an abusive parent.[2]

Adult survivors of childhood abuse often form intense, unstable relationships. Some find it very hard to tolerate being alone, but are also extremely wary of others. Terrified of being abandoned on the one hand, and of being dominated on the other, they fluctuate between extremes of submissiveness and rebellion. This has been termed 'sitting duck syndrome'.[3] In the most extreme cases, survivors of childhood abuse may find themselves involved in abuse of others, either in the role of passive bystander or, more rarely, as a perpetrator.

Assisting a child in overcoming abuse is a challenge, but children can and do overcome trauma. Helping children make sense of things by listening to them and acting on their behalf when necessary will make a lot of difference to their ability to recover from their childhood traumas. Apathy should not be tolerated by society, and it is part of the problem. A recent example of the way in which apathy itself can form part of the abuse is the sex abuse cases within the Catholic Church which began coming to light in the mid-1980s. The cases involved sexual abuse of minors by priests and received significant media attention. Sadly, cases occurring over many decades have since been reported in numerous countries throughout the world. Much of the scandal focused on members of the church's hierarchy who didn't report allegations of abuse to the civil authorities. In many cases they reassigned those accused to other locations, where they continued to have contact with minors.

Sociopathic relatives

It isn't just apathy but sociopathy itself that can be an entrenched problem within families. Siblings, grandparents, aunts and uncles may have some degree of sociopathy, or a related condition like narcissism. Nor is it uncommon for the children of sociopaths, whether or not they are sociopathic themselves, to attract, and be attracted to, sociopathic partners in later life. In this way the cycle of abuse can often be transferred from one generation to the next. And sometimes sociopaths join forces, or pair up with others with conditions of zero or limited empathy such as malignant narcissism. When these types combine they make for a potent and lethal mix. Such couplings can prove almost impossible to contend with in families.

However, there is some evidence that narcissistic behaviour can diminish with age; for instance, abusive fathers sometimes settle down and become seemingly decent grandfathers. Sociopaths, on the other hand, rarely if ever improve significantly with age, though they may seemingly become more subdued owing to a reduction in the opportunities they have to inflict harm.

Family members often become the targets of manipulation, one against the other, with the consequence that the family is destroyed by the destructive elements within. More often than not other members of the family fall into line, taking on the role and function that suit the sociopath best once the sociopathic transaction has been conducted and the Sociopath-Empath-Apath Triad set-up is in place. All too often the empath, the family member who is more perceptive and sees the situation for what it is, becomes the target of family hostility, eventually ending up either walking away or being expelled from the family group.

In this chapter and the previous one we have proposed ways to help people in such dramatic and painful circumstances, but additional support may be necessary. In the UK, guidelines on domestic abuse have been drawn up in recognition of the fact that emotional abuse is overlooked. The government aims to see more youngsters come forward and access the support they need – for example, speaking to someone about the abuse or contacting a helpline or a specialist service.

Currently in the UK, however, there is no specific criminal offence of domestic violence. The definition that refers to 'incidents of threatening behaviour, violence or abuse' was adopted in 2004, although some argue that police and prosecutors make too narrow an interpretation of the term. New guidance issued in 2013 acknowledges that abuse towards a partner can often encompass a variety of harms beyond the physical but may not go far enough by failing to encompass abuse between other members of a family. Nevertheless the Home Office widened the definition of domestic abuse in March 2013 to include those aged 16 and 17, as well as including a wider range of coercive or threatening behaviour.

As indicated above, domestic abuse is not only an issue for adults, but also for children and teenagers. Young people's formative years are difficult at the best of times, but a lack of experience in relationships and issues with self-confidence can mean they feel they have nowhere to turn. A myriad supportive networks and approaches are available (see the list of useful addresses and websites at the end of this book), although as each person's circumstances differ some forms of support are more helpful than others. Family therapy, for example, is unlikely to prove helpful when there is a sociopath is in the family, because sociopaths do not respond constructively to therapy and may run rings around the therapist, however well qualified and experienced he or she may be. On the other hand, the non-sociopathic members of the family or household may well need this kind of psychological support; it may prove highly beneficial to have someone outside the experience who is able to listen to their concerns.

But a word of caution: even trained and experienced counsellors and psychotherapists may not be *au fait* with the issue of sociopathic abuse. They may fail to appreciate the nuances of sociopathy and the abusive interactions that can occur in families where sociopaths lurk. Our advice is to ask prospective therapists about their experience of working with families and sociopathic abuse, and only to engage in this kind of support if you feel confident in the therapist's ability to work effectively with this complex family dynamic and to handle the situation well.

Since those with first-hand experience of sociopathic abuse began to promote awareness about sociopathy and its harms, a significant amount of help has become available and numerous support groups have been set up to assist those overcoming sociopathic abuse. However, these groups are intended for adults, *not* children, though young adults may also find them beneficial. At present, we are not aware of any groups that cater specifically for young children or teenagers. The issue of online support for children remains fraught with difficulties, a situation that acts as a deterrent to would-be groups and campaigners, not least because it is vital to protect children from the risk of further abuse.

Laying down the law with problem grandparents and other family members

If the sociopathic family member happens to be someone other than a parent, for example a grandparent, aunt or uncle, then the situation can be equally murky. Adults with sociopathic parents or siblings are likely to feel torn between their parents' and society's expectation that grandparents, aunts and uncles should have access to their grandchildren, grand-nieces and grand-nephews, and their desire to properly protect their child from abuse. Such parents also have to contend with their own experiences of emotional, physical or sexual abuse at the hands of their own parents or siblings, and this prior experience can ring alarm bells about abuse occurring to their own children if contact is maintained. This situation may prove just too difficult for the parents to deal with and may deter them from allowing their children to have any kind of relationship with the sociopathic family member.

In the case of sociopathic grandparents it is fairly common for the parents to allow the grandparents to begin a relationship with their grandchildren, hoping that things will be different this time, but unfortunately this is rarely the case: sociopathy is a lifelong and untreatable disorder. If contact is maintained, however, even in a limited way, the children involved may eventually be torn apart by the grief of having to sever a relationship with the unhealthy family member. And the parent is likely to experience secondary trauma if her children are abused by other members of the family. She may end up feeling mortified at having done more harm than good by allowing the sociopath access to her children.

It is important that parents consider the pros and cons of letting other family members have contact with, and access to, their children. In her helpful blog, 'Light's Blog at Light's House' (see 'Useful addresses' for details), Drew Keys suggests the following questions be used to provide help in the decision-making process. If the answer to the questions below is 'no', then a rule of no contact is probably safest and best:

- Is the previously abusive family member a very different person to you from the one you remember?
- Do you currently have a healthy, functional and stable relationship with the family member?

- Does the family member respect your choices and boundaries as a parent?
- Does the family member follow your requests about how you want your children to be treated and behave?
- Would you recommend your parent or other family member as babysitter to your best friend without any hesitation, and would you feel comfortable giving your word that the family member would never harm your friend's child?

If you find it very difficult to make a decision of this nature, seek professional help, as other family members will not be neutral or objective. Professionals may include an adviser from the local social services child protection department, a family therapist or a family lawyer.

In the UK grandparents have no automatic rights in respect of their grandchildren. Nor do aunts and uncles have any special rights. If family members wish to reinstate contact it may become necessary for them to obtain a court order. The implementation of the Children Act 1989 made it possible for the court to make a number of different orders in respect of children.

One of the most common types of court order is a **contact order**. This term has replaced the word 'access' but it is essentially the same thing. An applicant for an order of this type asks for the court to allow them to have either direct or indirect contact. **Direct contact** is where the person to whom the order is granted will be able to physically see the children and perhaps take part in activities with them. **Indirect contact** is where the person will talk to the child by letter, telephone, email and text messages. If one or both parents raise objections the grandparents will have to attend a full hearing in which both parties put forward their evidence. In light of this, the offending grandparent may occasionally continue to pursue this course of action for fear of his or true nature being exposed. If an abusive grandparent does continue to pursue a contact order, make sure any letters, emails or other indicators of abuse are kept as evidence for use in court.

The situation is similar in the USA. There is also no such thing as 'Grandparents' Rights' and a ruling made by the Supreme Court applies to all 50 states.[4] State courts considering non-parent visitation petitions must apply 'a presumption that fit parents act in the best interests of their children', and must give special weight to a fit parent's decision to deny non-parent visitation: 'Choices [parents make] about the upbringing of children . . . are among associational rights . . . sheltered by the Fourteenth Amendment against the State's unwarranted usurpation, disregard, or disrespect.' Grandparents may try to gain access, but 'fit' parents who have established no-contact boundaries may always block attempts to access their grandchildren.

What if you suspect your child has sociopathic traits?

Although those who have children with a sociopath can have healthy, happy offspring, unfortunately some people experience years of problems with their children. There may be a number of reasons for this: the sociopath may have abandoned the children and left the other parent to raise them alone; the children may have been used as a pawn in the sociopathic parent's manipulation games; or – and this is the worst scenario of all – the children may turn out to be sociopathic themselves. Here we turn to the issues facing the parents of sociopathic children.

Sociopathy in children is very much a hidden problem in society, but a few films have been made that draw attention to sociopathic children and allow us to glimpse the nature of the problem. The issue is the focus of the contentious US thriller *The Good Son* (1993).

The film was universally slated. Critics thought the sociopathic child, Henry, was too unrealistic, with one critic contending that 'This is a very evil little boy . . . what rings false is that the Macaulay Culkin character isn't really a little boy at all . . . His speech is much too sophisticated and ironic for that, and so is his reasoning and his cleverness . . . he seems more like a distasteful device by the filmmakers, who apparently think there is a market for glib one-liners by child sadists.'[5] Nevertheless, for those who live in close proximity to a sociopathic child, the film, with the exception of its implausible ending, is not so far-fetched; in fact the main character's glibness, artificiality and indifference are an accurate depiction of real-life child sociopathy. For example, here's a passage of dialogue from the film. A young boy called Mark Evans stays with his aunt and uncle and befriends his cousin Henry, who is the same age. But Henry begins showing increasing signs of sociopathic behaviour. Henry has thrown a plastic doll over a highway overpass into oncoming traffic, causing a massive pile-up:

MARK: Do you know what you did?

HENRY: Hey, come on. We did it together.

MARK: You could've killed people . . .

HENRY: . . . with your help . . .

MARK: Hey, I didn't know you were gonna do that!

HENRY: I feel sorry for you, Mark. You just don't know how to have fun.

MARK: What?

HENRY: It's because you're scared all the time. I know. I used to be scared too. But that was before I found out.

MARK: Found out what?

HENRY: That once you realize you can do anything . . . you're free. You could fly. Nobody can touch you . . . nobody. Mark . . . don't be afraid to fly.

MARK: You're sick . . .

The issue of child sociopathy is also the focus of the 2011 US/UK film *We Need to Talk about Kevin*. In the film we see the problems through the eyes of the mother, Eva, who is the 'seeing' person (the empath) in the family. Throughout her son Kevin's life (the sociopath) he has been detached and difficult. He does not bond with his mother and as a baby he cries incessantly, rebuffs her attempts at affection, and shows no interest in anything. While Kevin is still small, his mother Eva's frustration with his intractability drives her to him throw against the wall, breaking his arm. Eva's husband dismisses her concerns, makes excuses for his son, gives Kevin a bow and arrow set and teaches him archery. Kevin becomes an excellent marksman. There follows a series of disturbing accidents to the household. While the mother blames Kevin, the father insists that Kevin is blameless. Since her earlier concerns were dismissed, the mother keeps to herself her intensifying fear of her son. The story culminates with Kevin plotting and executing several multiple killings. The paradox is that no one other than his mother talks about Kevin or his disturbing behaviour. No one 'sees' the problem for what it is.

Callous unemotional traits

By the time a child with such tendencies (we hope not as extreme) reaches school age, he or she is already on the way to developing into a sociopath. She may interact well with school friends but the signs of anti-social behaviour are already there. Some children exert control over others by bullying them in the school playground while showing a different personality at home. They are therefore difficult to detect, a problem compounded by the fact that no psychiatrist or psychologist will label a child a sociopath because it is regarded only as a potential problem at that stage. Instead, if pushed, psychologists identify these children as having **conduct disorder** or **callous unemotional traits**. But more often than not, these children are not identified or brought to the attention of mental health professionals at all. Some may be passed off as anti-social and eventually get caught up within the criminal justice system, especially sociopathic boys.

All children make mistakes and have times when they are aggressive, lie and manipulate because these traits are part of human nature, but children with callous unemotional traits, conduct disorder or sociopathy display behaviour that is extreme. These children are capable of acts of great harm carried out with intent, as witnessed in our example of James the school bully. James showed no guilt about getting others to gang up on Sam, or attempting to end his 'favourite' teacher's career. Such children exist and are not the stuff of fiction; many have significant problems with aggression and deceit, and will manipulate their way out of situations. And, just like their adult counterparts, they seem to have no conscience about their actions or care about the consequences that befall others.

Identifying sociopathic children

Recently doctors have performed fMRI scans of the brains of children with callous unemotional traits, focusing on an area of the brain called the amygdala, the part of the brain where fear and negative emotions appear to be processed. In one recent study scientists showed children pictures of other people in emotionally distressing situations. Typically children have a strong amygdala response to other people's distress; however in this study it was found that children with callous unemotional traits showed no discernible amygdala response on fMRI scans when they observed other people in distressing situations. This is the first time such a study has been done involving children. It reflects what has been found in many other studies carried out on adult sociopaths, and the findings are changing researchers' perception of sociopathy. Some scientists now believe these traits result from an under-arousal of the amygdala in these children's brains.[6]

Most of us learn to care about how other people feel by seeing emotion and fear in them, which causes our own discomfort. If you don't feel discomfort or fear yourself, and you don't notice it in other people, you are highly unlikely to develop the higher-order human functions of empathy and moral conscience. As we stated in Chapter 1, sociopaths recognize that other people have feelings and emotions and use them to their advantage, but they don't feel much themselves. Anti-social children with callous unemotional traits appear to be disconnected from other people's emotions just like adult sociopaths. Identifying children with these traits early and getting them into treatment is crucial. By the time these children reach puberty, it's often too late and they are untreatable.

So what are the warning signs? The **Macdonald triad**, proposed by J. M. Macdonald in 1963 and also known as the triad of socio-pathy, is a set of three behavioural characteristics – animal cruelty, obsession with fire setting, and persistent bedwetting (past the age of five) – originally thought to be associated with later violent tendencies. However this particular combination of behaviours has not been properly validated and the characterization has been more or less debunked. Today, younger children whose disruptive and aggressive behaviour takes place within the home but whose problem behaviours do not meet the criteria for conduct disorder may be diagnosed as having **oppositional defiant disorder**.

The key features present in older children with conduct disorder or high callous unemotional traits vary in intensity and breadth, but hallmark tendencies include a lack of conscience, lack of empathy, and lying and manipulative behaviour. According to the Royal College of Psychiatrists, there is no single cause of conduct disorder but many different possible reasons which lead to the condition. Children may be more likely to develop an oppositional defiant disorder or conduct disorder if they:

- have certain genes leading to anti-social behaviour – boys are also more likely to have these disorders than girls;
- have difficulties learning good social and acceptable behaviour;

- have a difficult temperament;
- have learning or reading difficulties, making it difficult to understand and take part in lessons. It is then easy to get bored, feel
  stupid and misbehave;
- are depressed;
- have been bullied or abused;
- are 'hyperactive' – this causes difficulties with self-control,
  paying attention and following rules;
- are involved with other difficult young people and drug abuse.

In children with these traits, evidence suggests that there are
genetic and physiological elements to the problem, although our
understanding of the condition is still in its infancy. The problem
can also be exacerbated by the way the child interacts with his
social environment, including what behaviours he learns at home,
so in these ways the problem is perpetuated in families. It can be
extremely tough on the parents of children with sociopathic traits:
first, it is emotionally exhausting and shaming to deal with a child
that doesn't care about others; on top of that the family are likely
to have to cope with the resulting slurs and public humiliation.

What can be done?

So what if you are a mother or father with normal levels of empathy
and your child is showing clear signs of callous unemotional behaviour? Of all the sociopathic relations to contend with, this must
surely be the hardest, not least because options for both support
and treatment are severely limited. As we stated earlier, many boys
with sociopathic tendencies end up within the criminal justice
system, while girls with the condition often go undetected, their
behaviour put down to all manner of things including puberty. The
net result of failure to detect sociopathy in children and to have
effective responses to the problem in place is that the situation per-
petuates sociopathic parenting and the cycle of abuse.

   What we do know is that there is no point in disciplining a child
with sociopathic traits more severely. Children with these traits
seem to be completely unmoved by punishment and will repeat
the same sort of misbehaviour again. Therefore it is important
to appreciate that children with callous unemotional traits are
punishment insensitive; they are very reward-driven but fearless,
so they will not be prevented from doing harm or taking risks by

being chastised. Parents need as much support as can be mustered, though sadly this is rarely available. A formal referral to a child psychologist or psychiatrist could be beneficial for diagnostic purposes and treatment, but this option is not readily available.

Is there anything you can do? At present a study is being conducted which suggests that increased physical contact and improved eye contact between parents or carers and the child may make some difference to the severity of these traits over time. Little is known of the parent–child emotional bond in such cases, but there is some evidence to suggest that these callous unemotional features in children are not immutable. Studies have found that children exposed to lower levels of physical punishment showed decreases in callous unemotional traits over time, while higher levels of parental warmth and involvement (as reported by the child) led to decreases in both callous unemotional traits and antisocial behaviour.

The researchers involved in the current study advise parents to look their child in the eyes to see if they can persuade him to look back. While to most of us this seems a natural response, young children with callous unemotional traits rarely look their parents in the eyes. Researchers are optimistic that this intervention can bring about a real difference; they consider that if they can train young children to look at their parents in this way, they can change the children's development. But only time will tell whether there is merit in this approach.

Before we leave this topic we want to reaffirm a vital issue, and that is the importance of communication. Talking about the problem at home, at school, and among friends and relatives provides opportunities for early intervention. Not talking about it and ignoring it, hoping it will go away, may have disastrous consequences for all concerned. What we need to do is heed the message of the film *We Need to Talk about Kevin* and learn to talk about it.

8

End-stage recovery

The conflict between the will to deny horrible events and the will to proclaim them aloud is the central dialectic of psychological trauma.

(J. Lewis Herman)

Someone attempting to straighten out their life after a traumatic time with a sociopath may be excessively aware of sociopaths for some time afterwards. It may seem as if the entire world is populated with callous sociopaths, though this distorted view is usually only temporary. The situation occurs because the person's senses are working overtime, making her over-alert to danger. Luckily, this state of super-vigilance will eventually diminish. Nevertheless it is not uncommon during this period for people to purge themselves of all the parasitic and unwholesome individuals that have accumulated in their life over the years. The process, albeit anxious and turbulent, is also healthy and restorative. It is part of the transformation process and signifies the end phase of recovery. It stems from a desire to see wholesale change and the adoption of a new, stronger persona.

The process may involve making even more changes than you anticipated: a house move, a new job, seeking new horizons. On one hand this new state may lead to further alienation; a sense of having to 'go it alone'. Other people may not be going through a similar transformation process. They may struggle to come to terms with the changes in you, their friend, partner or colleague, which can further add to the sense of alienation, frustrations and sense of stigma felt by the person in recovery. On the other hand, the new situation feels good because it is indicative of your increased independence. Many people feel a newfound sense of freedom and confidence, and a greater awareness of 'self'.

The end stage of recovery is a time to be bold, a time to take risks and follow your instincts. It may involve lots of unexpected changes but eventually, with any luck, balance will be restored.

When it comes to new relations and friendships, someone betrayed in the ways discussed in this book may find themselves less trusting than before. The degree of mistrust will vary owing to your personality as well as the nature of the betrayal. But the crux of the matter is that under normal circumstances if a betrayal has occurred, the wrongdoer would be expected to admit that he or she has inflicted a deep hurt.

For people who have been traumatized by a sociopath, this circumstance is denied them. An apology will never be forthcoming, not a genuine one at any rate. So the person in recovery must contend with an inadequate ending to the whole sorry saga. With a sociopath there is no satisfying end point or sense of closure to the situation. The end stage of recovery may be a lone journey, but it is not one to be taken wearing a badge of shame. You must learn to walk tall, to cast off the stigma and social disapproval of experiencing trauma at the hands of another human being.

Dealing with stigma

The central dilemma for people recovering from sociopathic abuse, according to Judith Herman in her landmark book *Trauma and Recovery*, is whether to be vociferous or keep quiet about their past situation. One way of dealing with the stigma is to quietly get on with your life and not let others' views bother you. Another is to confront the stigma head on. It is up to each and every individual to deal with the issue as best suits him or her. For many adult children abused by a sociopathic parent, getting over the stigma of child abuse is the biggest challenge, one that may be met by not letting the experience adversely affect the rest of your life. It requires you to learn to love yourself and to accept your past experiences, good and bad. Hopefully at some point those nearing the end stages of recovery will reach a place where they recognize that while they were a victim of abuse as a child, they are surviving that abuse as an adult and managing their lives well.

Tackling the stigma of sociopathic abuse can be part of the end stage of recovery. Campaigning about the hidden harms of sociopathic abuse is one way of going about this. The self-help ethos of many recovery groups is not only an effective way of reaching out and supporting marginalized individuals and groups, but is also beneficial to society as a whole, as the act of coming together and taking collective action raises the profile of the issue and alters public perceptions. Moreover, by supporting campaigning groups or being vocal about sociopathic abuse, the abused person can come to appreciate his own journey and his movement through the process of recovery. For some, getting the issue out there in the public domain is an absolute necessity, a way of breaking the silence on the issue and challenging the apathy in society. However, what often stops people from speaking out about the problem is the shame inflicted upon them by the rest of society.

Jeremy Rifkin, author of *The Empathic Civilization*, describes a shaming culture as one that 'pretends to adhere to the highest possible standards of moral perfection'. Historically shaming cultures have been the most aggressive and violent because 'they lock up the empathic impulse'. We see this in the way that young women are said to be 'asking for it' when they are sexually assaulted, for example. This kind of response stops us from empathizing with their plight. Breaking down the stigma requires individual and collective activity to expose the harms of anti-social behaviour. Thereafter each of us needs to contribute to a culture where empathy exists as a prized virtue with the potential to transform human beings into highly social beings. Empathic responses can be learnt by means of cultural transmission. Parents, teachers, adults of all ages, should be the next generation's enlightened witnesses, helping children make emotional connections and advance social behaviour in society.

In his book Rifkin highlights a study that is worth recounting here. Having observed the behaviour of adolescent elephants in an animal park in South Africa, zoologists noted that for unknown reasons the elephants had begun to taunt and kill other animals. It was only when the zoologists recollected that, years earlier, they had culled the adult male elephants in order to ease overcrowding and decided to bring back to the park two older male elephants that order was reintroduced. It transpired that the reintroduction of the older male elephants stopped the younger elephants from behaving in an anti-social manner. Rifkin suggests that we humans, like the elephants in the study, require adult role models to set the boundaries on social behaviour. It is up to each and every one of us to set standards of social behaviour and maintain these by establishing clear boundaries.

Getting a child to understand how her behaviour affects other children and how she would feel if the same misbehaviour was enacted on her requires a parent or adult with a well-developed conscience and empathy. The adult's role is to act as the child's guide, helping the child reflect on her own behaviour, feel remorse and prepare to make reparation for her misdemeanour. Through this process the positive human attributes of social behaviour and empathy are advanced. The benefits are likely to be substantial. After all, as internationally renowned professor of psychiatry Stanley Greenspan argues: 'Mental health requires a feeling of connectedness with humanity . . . which in turn requires a well-developed sense of empathy.'

Appendix: The Empathy Quotient (EQ) test

The Empathy Quotient, devised by Simon Baron-Cohen, is intended to measure how easily you pick up on other people's feelings and how strongly you are affected by others' feelings. If you wish to take the test, read each of the 60 statements very carefully and rate how strongly you agree or disagree with them by circling your answer. If using the test reproduced in the table, work out your EQ score using the points system explained at the end of the questionnaire. Or you can perform the test online by visiting http://glennrowe. net/BaronCohen/EmpathyQuotient/EmpathyQuotient.aspx.

There are no right or wrong answers, or trick questions. We do not advise you take this test too seriously – it is provided here simply for your interest. A child version of the Empathy Quotient is available in Baron-Cohen, *Zero Degrees of Empathy: A New Theory of Human Cruelty* (2011), London: Allen Lane/Penguin Books, Appendix 1, 135–9.

The Empathy Quotient (EQ) test

1 I can easily tell if someone else wants to enter a conversation.	strongly agree	slightly agree	slightly disagree	strongly disagree
2 I prefer animals to humans.	strongly agree	slightly agree	slightly disagree	strongly disagree
3 I try to keep up with the current trends and fashions.	strongly agree	slightly agree	slightly disagree	strongly disagree
4 I find it difficult to explain to others things that I understand easily, when they don't understand it first time.	strongly agree	slightly agree	slightly disagree	strongly disagree
5 I dream most nights.	strongly agree	slightly agree	slightly disagree	strongly disagree
6 I really enjoy caring for other people.	strongly agree	slightly agree	slightly disagree	strongly disagree
7 I try to solve my own problems rather than discussing them with others.	strongly agree	slightly agree	slightly disagree	strongly disagree
8 I find it hard to know what to do in a social situation.	strongly agree	slightly agree	slightly disagree	strongly disagree

9 I am at my best first thing in the morning.	strongly agree	slightly agree	slightly disagree	strongly disagree
10 People often tell me that I went too far in driving my point home in a discussion.	strongly agree	slightly agree	slightly disagree	strongly disagree
11 It doesn't bother me too much if I am late meeting a friend.	strongly agree	slightly agree	slightly disagree	strongly disagree
12 Friendships and relationships are just too difficult, so I tend not to bother with them.	strongly agree	slightly agree	slightly disagree	strongly disagree
13 I would never break a law, no matter how minor.	strongly agree	slightly agree	slightly disagree	strongly disagree
14 I often find it difficult to judge if something is rude or polite.	strongly agree	slightly agree	slightly disagree	strongly disagree
15 In a conversation, I tend to focus on my own thoughts rather than on what my listener might be thinking.	strongly agree	slightly agree	slightly disagree	strongly disagree
16 I prefer practical jokes to verbal humour.	strongly agree	slightly agree	slightly disagree	strongly disagree
17 I live life for today rather than the future.	strongly agree	slightly agree	slightly disagree	strongly disagree
18 When I was a child, I enjoyed cutting up worms to see what would happen.	strongly agree	slightly agree	slightly disagree	strongly disagree
19 I can pick up quickly if someone says one thing but means another.	strongly agree	slightly agree	slightly disagree	strongly disagree
20 I tend to have very strong opinions about morality.	strongly agree	slightly agree	slightly disagree	strongly disagree
21 It is hard for me to see why some things upset people so much.	strongly agree	slightly agree	slightly disagree	strongly disagree
22 I find it easy to put myself in somebody else's shoes.	strongly agree	slightly agree	slightly disagree	strongly disagree
23 I think that good manners are the most important thing a parent can teach their child.	strongly agree	slightly agree	slightly disagree	strongly disagree
24 I like to do things on the spur of the moment.	strongly agree	slightly agree	slightly disagree	strongly disagree
25 I am good at predicting how someone will feel.	strongly agree	slightly agree	slightly disagree	strongly disagree
26 I am quick to spot when someone in a group is feeling awkward or uncomfortable.	strongly agree	slightly agree	slightly disagree	strongly disagree
27 If I say something that someone else is offended by, I think that that's their problem, not mine.	strongly agree	slightly agree	slightly disagree	strongly disagree

	strongly agree	slightly agree	slightly disagree	strongly disagree
28 If anyone asked me if I liked their haircut, I would reply truthfully, even if I didn't like it.	strongly agree	slightly agree	slightly disagree	strongly disagree
29 I can't always see why someone should have felt offended by a remark.	strongly agree	slightly agree	slightly disagree	strongly disagree
30 People often tell me that I am very unpredictable.	strongly agree	slightly agree	slightly disagree	strongly disagree
31 I enjoy being the centre of attention at any social gathering.	strongly agree	slightly agree	slightly disagree	strongly disagree
32 Seeing people cry doesn't really upset me.	strongly agree	slightly agree	slightly disagree	strongly disagree
33 I enjoy having discussions about politics.	strongly agree	slightly agree	slightly disagree	strongly disagree
34 I am very blunt, which some people take to be rudeness, even though this is unintentional.	strongly agree	slightly agree	slightly disagree	strongly disagree
35 I don't tend to find social situations confusing.	strongly agree	slightly agree	slightly disagree	strongly disagree
36 Other people tell me I am good at understanding how they are feeling and what they are thinking.	strongly agree	slightly agree	slightly disagree	strongly disagree
37 When I talk to people, I tend to talk about their experiences rather than my own.	strongly agree	slightly agree	slightly disagree	strongly disagree
38 It upsets me to see an animal in pain.	strongly agree	slightly agree	slightly disagree	strongly disagree
39 I am able to make decisions without being influenced by people's feelings.	strongly agree	slightly agree	slightly disagree	strongly disagree
40 I can't relax until I have done everything I had planned to do that day.	strongly agree	slightly agree	slightly disagree	strongly disagree
41 I can easily tell if someone else is interested or bored with what I am saying.	strongly agree	slightly agree	slightly disagree	strongly disagree
42 I get upset if I see people suffering on news programmes.	strongly agree	slightly agree	slightly disagree	strongly disagree
43 Friends usually talk to me about their problems as they say that I am very understanding.	strongly agree	slightly agree	slightly disagree	strongly disagree
44 I can sense if I am intruding, even if the other person doesn't tell me.	strongly agree	slightly agree	slightly disagree	strongly disagree
45 I often start new hobbies but quickly become bored with them and move on to something else.	strongly agree	slightly agree	slightly disagree	strongly disagree

46 People sometimes tell me that I have gone too far with teasing.	strongly agree	slightly agree	slightly disagree	strongly disagree
47 I would be too nervous to go on a big rollercoaster.	strongly agree	slightly agree	slightly disagree	strongly disagree
48 Other people often say that I am insensitive, though I don't always see why.	strongly agree	slightly agree	slightly disagree	strongly disagree
49 If I see a stranger in a group, I think that it is up to them to make an effort to join in.	strongly agree	slightly agree	slightly disagree	strongly disagree
50 I usually stay emotionally detached when watching a film.	strongly agree	slightly agree	slightly disagree	strongly disagree
51 I like to be very organized in day to day life and often make lists of the chores I have to do.	strongly agree	slightly agree	slightly disagree	strongly disagree
52 I can tune into how someone else feels rapidly and intuitively.	strongly agree	slightly agree	slightly disagree	strongly disagree
53 I don't like to take risks.	strongly agree	slightly agree	slightly disagree	strongly disagree
54 I can easily work out what another person might want to talk about.	strongly agree	slightly agree	slightly disagree	strongly disagree
55 I can tell if someone is masking their true emotion.	strongly agree	slightly agree	slightly disagree	strongly disagree
56 Before making a decision I always weigh up the pros and cons.	strongly agree	slightly agree	slightly disagree	strongly disagree
57 I don't consciously work out the rules of social situations.	strongly agree	slightly agree	slightly disagree	strongly disagree
58 I am good at predicting what someone will do.	strongly agree	slightly agree	slightly disagree	strongly disagree
59 I tend to get emotionally involved with a friend's problems.	strongly agree	slightly agree	slightly disagree	strongly disagree
60 I can usually appreciate the other person's viewpoint, even if I don't agree with it.	strongly agree	slightly agree	slightly disagree	strongly disagree

The EQ test was devised by Professor Simon Baron-Cohen and Dr Sally Wheelwright and first appeared in the following academic journals: *Journal of Autism and Developmental Disorders* (2004) 34, 163; *Psychological Medicine* (2004) 34, 911.

The EQ test is a questionnaire that is completed by adults (if over 16 years old) or by their parent (if using the child or adolescent version of this test). It reveals individual differences in empathy, both 'cognitive' and 'affective' empathy. It can be used for screening purposes but is not diagnostic. A low score indicates low empathy.

The EQ test is provided 'as is', and the creators and the university make no warranties of any kind, either express or implied, concerning the EQ. The EQ is provided for research use only and should not be used to inform clinical decisions. Any commercial use of the EQ is prohibited without the prior express written permission from the creators and the university.

How to work out your EQ score

Score **two points** for each of the following items if you answered 'strongly agree' or **one point** if you answered 'slightly agree': 1, 6, 19, 22, 25, 26, 35, 36, 37, 38, 41, 42, 43, 44, 52, 54, 55, 57, 58, 59, 60.

Score **two points** for each of the following items if you answered 'strongly disagree' or **one point** if you answered 'slightly disagree': 4, 8, 10, 11, 12, 14, 15,18, 21, 27, 28, 29, 32, 34, 39, 46, 48, 49, 50. *All other questions are not scored.*

What your score means

On average, most women score about 47 and most men about 42. Most people with Asperger syndrome or high-functioning autism score about 20.

0–32: you have a lower than average ability for understanding how other people feel and responding appropriately.

33–52: you have an average ability for understanding how other people feel and responding appropriately. You know how to treat people with care and sensitivity.

53–63: you have an above average ability for understanding how other people feel and responding appropriately. You know how to treat people with care and sensitivity.

64–80: you have a very high ability for understanding how other people feel and responding appropriately. You know how to treat people with care and sensitivity.

Useful addresses

United Kingdom

Association of Shared Parenting: website: www.sharedparenting.org.uk
A membership organization with branches in Birmingham, Coventry and
Leicester; for details write to: Spring Cottage, Binton Hill, Stratford-upon-
Avon CV37 9TN

British Association of Counselling and Psychotherapy: tel.: 01455
883300; website: www.bacp.co.uk

The Centre for Separated Families: Coppergate House, 16 Brune Street,
London E1 7NJ; website: www.separatedfamilies.info

ChildLine: tel.: 0800 1111; website: www.childline.org.uk

If you think a child is in immediate danger and you live in the UK,
contact the police on emergency number 999 or call the NSPCC on
0808 800 5000. If you suspect a child may be at risk but not in imminent
danger, contact your local children's social services.

The Custody Minefield: contact details via website: www.thecustody
minefield.com

Equal Parenting Alliance: For immediate assistance call 0790 550 2856;
otherwise email via website: www.equalparentingalliance.com

Families Need Fathers: helpline 0300 0300 363, 7 a.m. to midnight daily;
website www.fnf.org.uk

Family Law Society: contact details only available via website: www.
familylawsociety.org. A gender-neutral organization founded in 2004 to
help families who are experiencing the pain of parental separation.

Fathers 4 Justice: general enquiries only via email from the website:
www.fathers-4-justice.org

Mind infoline: 0300 123 3393; website: www.mind.org.uk

National Society for Children and Family Contact: email contact only
via website: www.nscfc.com

National Society for Prevention of Cruelty to Children (NSPCC):
tel.: 0808 800 5000; website: www.nspcc.org.uk

Parents4Protest: contact details available only via website:
www.parents4protest.co.uk

UK Council for Psychotherapy: tel.: 020 7014 9955; website:
www.psychotherapy.org.uk

UK ManKind: website: www.mankind.org.uk. A website for male survivors of domestic abuse.

United Kingdom Psychological Trauma Society (formerly the **UK Trauma Group**): tel.: 07979 994057; website: wwwukpts.co.uk

Women's Aid: tel.: 0808 2000 247; website: www.womensaid.org.uk

United States of America

Alliance for Non-Custodial Parents Rights: website: http://ancpr.com A site producing information on various issues, including parental rights. Their *Winning Strategies Handbook* is available to download.

American Coalition for Fathers and Children: tel.: 800 978-3237 for general enquiries (very busy switchboard); website: www.acfc.org

Domestic Abuse Helpline for Men and Women (DAHMW): tel.: 1-888-7HELPLINE (1-888-743-5754); website: http://dahmw.org

Find a Psychologist: website: www.findapsychologist.org/about.html. Online resource with freely available directory of 11,000 psychologists with their credentials.

National Child Abuse Hotline: tel.: 1-800-4-A-CHILD (1-800-422-4453); website: www.childhelp.org

National Domestic Violence Hotline: tel.: 1-800-799-SAFE (7233); website: www.thehotline.org. This hotline provides advice, support and referral to battered women's shelters in your area.

Separated Parenting Access and Resource Center: website: www. deltabravo.net. A non-profit website-based organization with the aim of enabling children of divorcees to have access to both parents.

Canada

National Domestic Violence Hotline: tel.: 1-800-363-9010

Post-Traumatic Stress Disorder (PTSD) Association: contact available only by email via the website: ptsdassociation.com . Linkages with appropriate services, facilitation of research and discovery into the causation and effective treatment strategies for post-traumatic stress disorder.

Australia

National Lifeline: tel.: 131 114 (for crisis services in each Australian state)

National Sexual Assault, Family and Domestic Violence Counselling Line: tel.: 1800 737 732 (24 hours) or 1800RESPECT

One in Three Campaign: contact available only by email via the website: www.oneinthree.com.au. (One in three victims of family violence is male.)

International

International Directory of Domestic Violence Agencies: http://www. hotpeachpages.net. A global list of helplines and crisis centres.

World Wide Web

Aftermath: Surviving Psychopathy Foundation: contact by email via the website: www.aftermath-surviving-psychopathy.org or write to PO Box 267, Yorkville, IL 60560, USA

Anxiety Help Center: website: www.helpguide.org/topics/anxiety.htm. A site run by a non-profit group; no personal advice but useful resources are provided.

Bully OnLine: website: www.bullyonline.org. The world's largest resource on workplace bullying and related issues.

The Culture of Empathy: website: http://cultureofempathy.com. A portal for resources about the values of empathy and compassion worldwide.

EMDR Institute Inc.: website: www.emdr.com. Eye Movement Desensitization and Reprocessing is a treatment approach for trauma victims.

Emotional Health Help Center: website: www.helpguide.org/topics/ emotional_health.htm

Estranged Stories: website: www.estrangedstories.com. A site where people experiencing estrangement or cut off from their family can find support.

Facebook: website: www.facebook.com. Search using the terms 'sociopath' or 'narcissist' or 'psychopath' for survivor support groups. Some groups are closed and you have to request to join to become a member, while others are open forums available to anyone.

Light's Blog at Light's House: website: http://lightshouse.org/ lights-blog/#axzz1tQfINot0

Stress Help Center: website: www.helpguide.org/topics/stress.htm

References

1 Introduction: what the book is about

1   K. L. Barry, M. F. Fleming, L. B. Manwell and L. A. Copeland (1997), 'Conduct disorder and antisocial personality in adult primary care patients', *Journal of Family Practice* 45:2, 15–18. There is also an earlier study: J. F. Samuels, G. Nestadt, A. J. Romanoski, M. F. Folstein and P. R. McHugh (1994), 'DSM-III personality disorders in the community', *American Journal of Psychiatry* 151:7, 1055–62. This gave a prevalence estimate of 5.9 per cent of all types of personality disorders in adults in the community.

2   P. Babiak and R. D. Hare (2006), *Snakes in Suits*, New York: Collins.

3   J. Clarke (2009), *Working with Monsters: How to Identify and Protect Yourself from the Workplace Psychopath*, Sydney Australia: Random House.

4   J. W. Coid, M. Yang, S. Ullrich, A. Roberts and R. D. Hare (2009), 'Prevalence and correlates of psychopathic traits in the household population of Great Britain', *International Journal of Law and Psychiatry* 32, 265–73.

5   R. D. Hare (1993), *Without Conscience: The Disturbing World of the Psychopaths Among Us*, New York: Guilford Press, 83–96.

6   The term derives from Narcissus, the figure from Greek mythology known for his beauty. Narcissus was exceptionally proud and vain. Nemesis (the goddess of divine retribution or revenge) saw this characteristic in him and lured Narcissus to a pool where he saw his own reflection in the water. Not realizing it was an image of himself he soon fell in love with it, but unable to leave the beauty of his own reflection, he died.

7   P. Pinel (1801), *A Treatise on Insanity*, trans. D. D. Davies, 1806. Republished 1962, New York: Hafner, 150–6.

8   J. C. Pritchard (1835), *A Treatise on Insanity*, London: Sherwood, Gilbert and Piper. He also published (1847) *On the Different Forms of Insanity in Relation to Jurisprudence*, London: Hippolyte Bailliere.

9   R. D. Hare (1993), *Without Conscience*, New York: Guilford Press, 23–4.

10 S. Baron-Cohen (2011), *Zero Degrees of Empathy: A New Theory of Human Cruelty*, London: Allen Lane/Penguin Books. A full explanation of the empathy circuit can be found on pp. 19–28 of his book.

11 The emerging science on empathy is effectively conveyed in C. Keysers (2011), *The Empathic Brain: How the Understanding of Mirror Neurons Changes our Understanding of Human Nature*, Amsterdam: Social Brain Press.

3 A profile of the sociopath

1   Passive-aggressive behaviour takes many forms but can generally be described as a non-verbal aggression. It presents when one person is angry with another but does not or cannot tell them. Instead of communicating honestly when they feel upset, annoyed, irritated or disappointed such people shut off verbally, give angry looks, become obstructive or sulky. It can either be covert (concealed and hidden) or overt (blatant and obvious).

2   A. Harrn (2011), *What is Passive Aggressive Behaviour?*, Counselling Directory. Available at <www.counselling-directory.org.uk/counsellor-articles/ what-is-passive-aggressive-behaviour>.

3   H. B. Braiker (2004) *Who's Pulling Your Strings? How to Break the Cycle of Manipulation,* New York: McGraw-Hill.

4   P. Babiak and R. Hare (2006), *Snakes in Suits: When Psychopaths Go to Work*, New York: HarperCollins.

5   For more about pathological lying see C. C. Dike (2008), 'Pathological lying: symptom or disease?' *Psychiatric Times* 25, 7. Available at <www.psychiatrictimes.com/print/article/10168/1162950>.

6   S. Baron-Cohen (2011), *Zero Degrees of Empathy: A New Theory of Human Cruelty*, London: Allen Lane/Penguin Books.

7   M. K. F. Kreis and D. J. Cooke (2011), 'Capturing the psychopathic female: a prototypicality analysis of the Comprehensive Assessment of Psychopathic Personality (CAPP) across gender', *Behavioral Sciences and the Law* 29, 634–48. Also C. Logan (2011), 'La femme fatale: the female psychopath in fiction and clinical practice', *Mental Health Review Journal* 16:3, 118–27.

8   T. L. Nicholls, J. R. Ogloff, J. Brink and A. Spidel (2005), 'Psychopathy in women: a review of its clinical usefulness for assessing risk for aggression and criminality', *Behavioral Sciences and the Law* 23:6, 779–802.

4 Interactions of the sociopath

1   'The Perils of Obedience' as it appeared in *Harper's Magazine*. Available at <www.age-of-the-sage.org/psychology/milgram_perils_authority_1974.html>. The article was abridged and adapted from Stanley Milgram (1974), *Obedience to Authority.*

2   L. Gibson (2006), 'Mirrored emotions', *University of Chicago Magazine* 98, 4.

3   P. Salovey and J. D. Mayer (1990), 'Emotional intelligence', *Imagination, Cognition, and Personality* 9, 185–211.

4   C. Steiner and P. Perry (1997), *Achieving Emotional Literacy*, London: Bloomsbury, 11.

5   C. Louis de Canonville (2011), *The Effects of Gaslighting in Narcissistic Victim Syndrome*. Available online at <narcissisticbehavior.net/the-effects-of-gaslighting-in-narcissistic-victim-syndrome>.

6   R. Stern (2007), *The Gaslight Effect: How to Spot and Survive the Hidden Manipulation Others Use to Control Your Life*, New York: Morgan Road Books.

5 Coping in the aftermath of a destructive relationship

1   J. Bradshaw (1988), *Healing the Shame that Binds You*, Florida: Health Communications.
2   A. Miller (2007), *The Drama of the Gifted Child: The Search for the True Self*, revised edition, New York: Basic Books.
3   E. Kübler-Ross and D. Kessler (2007), *On Grief and Grieving: Finding the Meaning of Grief Through the Five Stages of Loss*, New York: Scribner.
4   The tips and strategies in this chapter are adapted from a guide on anger management by L. Garratt and P. Blackburn (2007), Newcastle Primary Care Trust, Newcastle, UK.
5   Available at <www.mind.org.uk>.
6   J. Lewis Herman (1992), 'Complex PTSD: A Syndrome in Survivors of Prolonged and Repeated Trauma', *Journal of Traumatic Stress* 5:3, 377–91.
7   B. P. R. Gersons (2005), 'Coping with the aftermath of trauma', *British Medical Journal* 330, 1038.
8   L. Shengold (1989), *Soul Murder: The Effects of Childhood Abuse and Deprivation*, New Haven: Yale University Press.

7 Dealing with complex family situations

1   R. Gardner (1998), *The Parent Alienation Syndrome: A Guide for Mental Health and Legal Professionals*, Cresskill, NJ: Creative Therapeutics.
2   J. Lewis Herman (1992), 'Complex PTSD: A Syndrome in Survivors of Prolonged and Repeated Trauma', *Journal of Traumatic Stress* 5:3, 377–91.
3   R. P. Kluft (1990), 'Incest and subsequent revictimization: The case of therapist–patient sexual exploitation, with a description of the sitting duck syndrome', in *Incest–Related Syndromes of Adult Psychopathology*, Washington, DC: American Psychiatric Press, 263–89.
4   US Supreme Court Case, *Troxel vs. Granville* (2000).
5   R. Ebert, 'The Good Son', *Chicago Sun-Times*, 24 September 1993.
6   M. R. Dadds and T. Rhodes (2008), 'Aggression in young children with concurrent callous–unemotional traits: can the neurosciences inform progress and innovation in treatment approaches?', *Philosophical Transactions of the Royal Society B: Biological Sciences* 363:1503, 2567–76.

Further reading and resources

Books

Anderson, D., *Love Fraud: How Marriage to a Sociopath Fulfilled My Spiritual Plan*. New Jersey: Anderly Publishing, 2010.

Babiak, P. and Hare, R. D., *Snakes in Suits: When Psychopaths Go to Work*. New York: Collins, 2006.

Baron-Cohen, S., *Zero Degrees of Empathy: A New Theory of Human Cruelty*. London: Allen Lane/Penguin Books, 2011.

Behary, W. T., *Disarming the Narcissist: Surviving and Thriving with the Self-Absorbed*. Oakland, CA: New Harbinger, 2008.

Bentley, B., *A Dance with the Devil: A True Story of Marriage to a Psychopath*. New York: Berkley Books, 2008.

Bradshaw, J., *Healing the Shame that Binds You*. Florida: Health Communications, 1988.

Bradshaw, J., *The Family: A New Way of Creating Solid Self-Esteem*. Florida: Health Communications, 1996.

Braiker, H. B., *Who's Pulling Your Strings? How to Break the Cycle of Manipulation and Regain Control of Your Life*. New York: McGraw-Hill, 2004.

Brown, N. W., *The Destructive Narcissistic Pattern*. Westport, CT: Praeger, 1998.

Brown, N. W., *Children of the Self-Absorbed*. Oakland, CA: New Harbinger, 2001.

Buttafuoco, M. J., *Getting it Through My Thick Skull*. Florida: Health Communications, 2009.

Clarke, J., *Working with Monsters: How to Identify and Protect Yourself From the Workplace Psychopath*. Sydney, Australia: Random House, 2009.

Covey, S. K., *In the Arms of a Sociopath*. Frederick, MD: PublishAmerica, 2009.

Daynes, K. and Fellows, J., *The Devil You Know: Looking Out for the Psycho in Your Life*. London: Coronet, 2011.

de Becker, G., *The Gift of Fear: Survival Signals That Protect Us From Violence*. Canada: Little, Brown, 1997.

Donaldson-Pressman, S. and Pressman, R. D., *Narcissistic Family: Diagnosis and Treatment*. New York: Wiley & Sons, 1997.

Dryden, W., *How to Accept Yourself*. London: Sheldon Press, 1999.

Engel, B., *The Jekyll and Hyde Syndrome: What to Do If Someone in Your Life Has a Dual Personality – or If You Do*. New Jersey: Wiley & Sons, 2007.

Evans, P., *Controlling People: How to Recognize, Understand, and Deal With People Who Try to Control You*. Canada: Adams Media, 2002.

Faulks, S., *Engleby*. London: Vintage, 2008.

Forward, S., *Toxic Parents: Overcoming Their Hurtful Legacy and Reclaiming Your Life*. New York: Bantam, 1989.

Golomb, E., *Trapped in the Mirror*. New York: Morrow, 1992.

Gootnick, I., *Why You Behave in Ways You Hate: And What You Can Do About It*. Roseville, CA: Penmarin Books, 1997.

Greenspan, S. L., with Benderly, B. L., *The Growth of the Mind and the Endangered Origins of Intelligence*. Reading, MA: Addison-Wesley, 1997.

Hare, R. D., *Without Conscience: The Disturbing World of the Psychopaths Among Us*. New York: Guilford Press, 1993.

Herbert, C. and Westmore, A., *Overcoming Traumatic Stress: A Self-help Guide Using Cognitive Behavioural Techniques*. London: Constable & Robinson, 2008.

Keysers, C., *The Empathic Brain: How the Understanding of Mirror Neurons Changes our Understanding of Human Nature*. Amsterdam: Social Brain Press, 2011.

Lerner, R., *The Object of My Affection is in My Reflection: Narcissists and Their Relationships*. Florida: Health Communications, 2009.

Lewis Herman, J., *Trauma and Recovery: The Aftermath of Violence – from Domestic Abuse to Political Terror*. New York: Basic Books, 1997.

McBride, K., *Will I Ever Be Good Enough? Healing the Daughters of Narcissistic Mothers*. New York: Simon & Schuster, 2008.

Miller, A., *For Your Own Good: Hidden Cruelty in Childrearing and the Roots of Violence*. New York: Farrar, Straus & Giroux, 1990.

Miller, A., *Banished Knowledge: Facing Childhood Injuries*. New York: Anchor Press, new edition 1997.

Miller, A., *Thou Shalt Not Be Aware: Society's Betrayal of the Child*. New York: Farrar, Straus and Giroux, 1998.

Miller, A., *The Truth Will Set You Free: Overcoming Emotional Blindness and Finding Your True Adult Self*. New York: Basic Books, 2001.

Miller, A., *The Body Never Lies: The Lingering Effects of Cruel Parenting*. New York: W. W. Norton, 2005.

Miller, A., *The Drama of the Gifted Child: The Search for the True Self*. New York: Basic Books, revised edition 2007.

Payson, E. D., *The Wizard of Oz and other Narcissists: Coping with the One-Way Relationship in Work, Love and Family*. Royal Oak, MI: Julian Day, 2002.

Rifkin, J., *The Empathic Civilization: The Race to Global Consciousness in a World in Crisis*. Cambridge: Polity Press, 2009.

Roan, C., *The Sociopath and Me*. Bloomington, IN: Trafford Publishing, 2011.

Ronson, J., *Out of the Ordinary: True Tales of Everyday Craziness*. London: Picador, 2006.

Ronson, J., *What I Do: More True Tales of Everyday Craziness*. London: Picador, 2007.

Ronson, J., *The Psychopath Test*. London: Picador, 2011.

Schiraldi, G., *The Post-Traumatic Stress Disorder Sourcebook: A Guide to Healing, Recovery and Growth*. New York: McGraw-Hill, 2009.

Silberschatz, G., *Transformative Relationships*. New York: Taylor & Francis, 2005.

Sichel, M., *Healing from Family Rifts*. New York: McGraw-Hill, 2004.

Simon, G., *In Sheep's Clothing*. Little Rock: Parkhurst Brothers, 1996.

Stern, R., *The Gaslight Effect: How to Spot and Survive the Hidden Manipulation Others Use to Control Your Life*. New York: Morgan Road Books, 2007.

Stout, M., *The Sociopath Next Door*. New York: Broadway Books, 2005.

Walker, M., *Surviving Secrets*. Buckingham: Open University Press, 2000.

Films

The Good Son (1993). American thriller directed by Joseph Ruben and written by English novelist Ian McEwan. The film stars Macaulay Culkin and Elijah Wood.

The Wave (German: *Die Welle*, 2008). A German film directed by Dennis Gansel. It is based on the book *The Wave*, which was inspired by the social experiment the Third Wave.

We Need to Talk about Kevin (2011). British-American film adapted and directed by Lynne Ramsay from US author Lionel Shriver's 2003 novel of the same name.

Index